Plant-Based Diet for Beginners

The Ultimate Guide for Beginners to a Whole-Food Vegan Diet to Eat Healthy, Lose Weight and Live Well

90+ Plant-Based Recipes with Pictures & 21-Day Meal Plan Included

Michael Gill

To all health enthusiasts
excited to embrace the Plant-Based Lifestyle

For the Planet, for the animals and for Yourself!

Table of Contents

CHAPTER 1: WHY GO PLANT-BASED? 11

BENEFITS OF THE PLANT-BASED DIET 11

BOOSTING THE IMMUNE SYSTEM WHEN ON THE PLANT-BASED EATING PLAN AND THROUGH

SUPPLEMENTATION 14

CHAPTER 2: THE BASICS OF A PLANT-BASED DIET 17

WHAT IS A PLANT-BASED DIET? 17

WHY YOU NEED TO CUT BACK ON PROCESSED AND ANIMAL-BASED PRODUCTS 19

PLANT-BASED DIET VS. VEGAN 21

GETTING STARTED ON A WHOLE FOOD 22

GETTING TO THE ROOT OF A PLANT-BASED DIET 24

CHAPTER 3: WHAT YOU STAND TO GAIN FROM A PLANT-BASED DIET 27

CHAPTER 4: THE MACRO AND MICRO ESSENTIALS OF A PLANT-BASED DIET ... 31

MACRONUTRIENTS 33

MICRONUTRIENTS 34

CHAPTER 5: HOW TO ELIMINATE BAD EATING HABITS 36

CHAPTER 6: PLANNING AND STOCKING YOUR PANTRY 45

BASIC SHOPPING LIST 48

CHAPTER 7: PLANT-BASED FOODS THAT BOOST YOUR IMMUNITY 52

KIWIS 52

BLUEBERRIES AND OTHER BERRIES 52

BROCCOLI AND OTHER CRUCIFEROUS VEGETABLES 53

GINGER 53

GREEN TEA 53

FOODS THAT HINDER THE IMMUNE SYSTEM 54

FOODS TO AVOID WITH AN AUTOIMMUNE DISEASE 55

A<small>RTIFICIAL</small> S<small>WEETENERS</small> 56

E<small>NVIRONMENTAL</small> R<small>ISKS</small> 57

CHAPTER 8:10 PLANT-BASED BEAUTY TREATMENTS TO USE ON YOUR SKIN

RECIPES.. **59**

A<small>VOCADO</small> 59

C<small>OCONUT</small> 59

R<small>AW</small> H<small>ONEY</small> 59

L<small>EMON</small> J<small>UICE</small> 60

A<small>PPLE</small>-C<small>IDER</small> V<small>INEGAR</small> 61

S<small>TRAWBERRIES</small> 61

B<small>ANANAS</small> 62

A<small>LMONDS AND</small> O<small>ATS</small> 62

O<small>LIVE</small> O<small>IL</small> 62

A<small>LOE</small> V<small>ERA</small> 63

CHAPTER 9:BREAKFASTS **64**

1. Tasty Oatmeal Muffins 64

2. Omelette with Chickpea Flour 64

3. White Sandwich Bread 65

4. A Toast to Remember 65

5. Tasty Panini 66

6. Tasty Oatmeal and Carrot Cake 66

7. Onion & Mushroom Tart with a Nice Brown Rice Crust 67

8. Perfect Breakfast Shake 68

9. Beet Gazpacho 68

10. Vegetable Rice 69

11. Courgette Risotto 69

12. Country Breakfast Cereal 70

13. Oatmeal Fruit Shake 70

14.   Amaranth Banana Breakfast Porridge 71

15.   Green Ginger Smoothie 71

16.   Orange Dream Creamsicle 71

17.   Strawberry Limeade 72

18.   Peanut Butter and Jelly Smoothie 72

19.   Banana Almond Granola 72

CHAPTER 10: SOUPS, SALADS, AND SIDES **73**

20.   Spinach Soup with Dill and Basil 73

21.   Coconut Watercress Soup 73

22.   Roasted Red Pepper and Butternut Squash Soup 74

23.   Tomato Pumpkin Soup 74

24.   Cauliflower Spinach Soup 75

25.   Avocado Mint Soup 75

26.   Creamy Squash Soup 76

27.   Cucumber Edamame Salad 76

28.   Best Broccoli Salad 77

29.   Rainbow Orzo Salad 77

30.   Broccoli Pasta Salad 78

31.   Eggplant & Roasted Tomato Farro Salad 78

32.   Garden Patch Sandwiches on Multigrain Bread 79

33.   Garden Salad Wraps 79

34.   Marinated Mushroom Wraps 80

35.   Tamari Toasted Almonds 80

36.   Nourishing Whole-Grain Porridge 81

37.   Pungent Mushroom Barley Risotto 81

CHAPTER 11: ENTRÉES **82**

38. Black Bean Dip...82

39. Cannellini Bean Cashew Dip...82

40. Cauliflower Popcorn...83

41. Cinnamon Apple Chips with Dip...83

42. Crunchy Asparagus Spears..84

43. Cucumber Bites with Chive and Sunflower Seeds.....................................85

44. Garlicky Kale Chips...85

45. Hummus-stuffed Baby Potatoes...86

46. Homemade Trail Mix...86

47. Nut Butter Maple Dip...86

48. Oven Baked Sesame Fries...87

49. Pumpkin Orange Spice Hummus..87

50. Quick English Muffin Mexican Pizzas..88

51. Quinoa Trail Mix Cups..88

CHAPTER 12: SMOOTHIES AND BEVERAGES 89

52. Fruity Smoothie...89

53. Energizing Ginger Detox Tonic...89

54. Warm Spiced Lemon Drink..90

55. Soothing Ginger Tea Drink..90

56. Nice Spiced Cherry Cider..90

57. Fragrant Spiced Coffee...91

58. Tangy Spiced Cranberry Drink...91

59. Warm Pomegranate Punch...92

60. Rich Truffle Hot Chocolate..92

61. Ultimate Mulled Wine..93

62. Pleasant Lemonade..93

63. Pineapple, Banana & Spinach Smoothie..94

64. Kale & Avocado Smoothie 94

65. Coconut & Strawberry Smoothie 94

66. Pumpkin Chia Smoothie 95

67. Cantaloupe Smoothie Bowl 95

68. Berry & Cauliflower Smoothie 95

69. Green Mango Smoothie 96

70. Chia Seed Smoothie 96

71. Mango Smoothie 96

SNACKS AND DESSERTS **97**

72. Mango And Banana Shake 97

73. Avocado Toast With Flaxseeds 97

74. Avocado Hummus 98

75. Plant Based Crispy Falafel 98

76. Waffles With Almond Flour 99

77. Mint & Avocado Smoothie 99

78. Simple Banana Fritters 100

79. Coconut And Blueberries Ice Cream 100

80. Peach Crockpot Pudding 100

81. Raspberries & Cream Ice Cream 101

82. Healthy Chocolate Mousse 101

83. Coconut Rice With Mangos 102

84. Nori Snack Rolls 102

85. Risotto Bites 103

86. Jicama and Guacamole 103

87. Curried Tofu "Egg Salad" Pitas 104

88. Garden Salad Wraps 104

89. Tamari Toasted Almonds 105

90. Avocado And Tempeh Bacon Wraps 105

91. Kale Chips 106

21-DAY MEAL PLAN **107**

CONCLUSIONS **109**

Chapter 1: Why Go Plant-Based?

As someone who was once in your shoes, I know that changing the way you eat can seem daunting. But keep in mind that this way of eating is not about what you can't eat; it's about all the delicious, nutritious foods you can eat. My goal with this book is to empower you to enjoy all the benefits of a whole-food, plant-based diet. So before we dive into the recipes, let's take a closer look at what exactly a whole-food, plant-based diet is and why it's so great.

Benefits of the Plant-Based Diet

When making the switch over to the plant-based eating plan, there are a number of benefits that come to mind. While these benefits are not immediate, they do manifest themselves in a relatively short period of time. As such, patience is an important key when looking to get the most out of this new dietary approach.

We are going to explore the benefits that come with the plant-based eating plan and how you can take full advantage of such benefits. Most importantly, you can find a great set of benefits which have the possibility of changing your life significantly.

Weight Loss

The most common reason why folks make this switch is for the purpose of losing weight. Truthfully, there is a great deal of logic in making this switch for the purpose of losing weight. Many individuals try their hardest to lose weight, yet they seem to come up short. And, while there are many factors that go into losing weight, the fact of the matter is that often there is a need to make a radical switch in eating habits.

The reasoning behind this lies in the functioning of the metabolism. The consumption of certain types of food, especially processed ones, creates a condition in which the body is unable to digest foods in the same manner.

For example, when you consume too much dairy, sugar and refined carbohydrates, your body quickly ships them off to fat storage. You would need to do massive amounts of exercise before you actually are able to tap into the body's fat reserves. Then, when you decide to cut down on the consumption of these foods, but not altogether, you end up causing your body to become confused.

To compound the issue, eating meat tends to slow down your metabolism as it takes much longer to digest meats, especially red meat, than it does to digest and process plant-based foods. As a result, you don't see the results you'd like to see.

When you switch over to the plant-based eating plan, you drastically alter your diet by cutting out the elements which slow down your metabolism. In return, your metabolism gets a break and progressively begins to speed up. In a manner of speaking, you are lightening the load on your metabolism as opposed to increasing it.

As your metabolism begins to speed up, you're able to digest foods faster and begin to accelerate the rate at which calories and nutrients are absorbed. Moreover, since plant-based foods don't accrue fat and calories like meat and processed foods do, then there is a definite advantage to boost weight loss. At the end of the day, consuming a great deal of plant-based foods makes a lot more sense if you're looking to lose weight.

Managing Illnesses

First, a bit of a disclaimer: if you are dealing with any medical condition, it is always a good idea to check with your doctor before making the switch. It might be that you have some type of dietary restriction that may interfere with the plant-based eating plan. While this is rather unusual, it's always a good idea to be sure you are not inadvertently putting yourself at risk.

That being said, managing illnesses becomes a lot easier once you go on the plant-based eating plan. In short, the plant-based eating plan looks to maximize the nutrition that you get from the foods you consume. By taking away meats, especially processed ones, and substituting it for fresh fruits and vegetables, you're actually doing your body a favor by helping it recover and regenerate.

However, there's one important secret that you might not be aware of. There are certain foods that we are allergic to, yet we don't even know how they are affecting us. In general, these are deep-fried, highly processed foods. In addition, sugary foods and drinks can do a number on your metabolism and immune system.

The fact of the matter is that a lot of foods that we consume on a regular basis contain large amounts of oils and carbohydrates. These ingredients tend to cause inflammation in the body. Now, inflammation is a logical response to the body as it tries to isolate a damaged part. By isolating a part that has been hurt or at least the body thinks it's hurt, you cause all kinds of inflammation throughout your body. This causes the brain to release a series of hormones and chemicals that trigger a stress response in your body. This further complicates things are inflammation in your digestive tract will cause you to have trouble absorbing nutrients. In short, you're eating and feeling full, but you're not actually getting any nutrition. When this process occurs, you are essentially asking for trouble.

By embracing the plant-based eating plan, you are giving your body the tools it needs to repair itself. By taking away potentially toxic elements, you're enabling your immune system to repair the body and thereby help alleviate some of the worse symptoms of whatever condition you may have. While going on this dietary approach is not going to cure what ails you, it will certainly help you manage the symptoms better and enable a better quality of life.

Muscle Growth and Fitness

One of the biggest concerns for athletes centers around the plant-based eating plan providing enough nutrients and protein, especially for demanding exercise routines. The short answer is that yes, the plant-based eating plan can provide athletes with all the nutrition they need. However, they need to do it the right way.

Now, it should be noted that most athletes are concerned about loading on protein especially if they are looking to bulk up. This is particularly true in the case of bodybuilders. In such cases, it's best to consume an additional protein supplement that can help provide the necessary protein load for building muscle.

However, beyond the rigorous requirements that bodybuilders have, regular folks and athletes need not be worried. The fact of the matter is that the plant-based eating plan provides ample room for protein so long as it's consumed on a regular basis. For instance, nuts provide a good deal of protein and healthy fats. Of course, we're not advocating that you must consume large amounts of nuts. Still, consuming a healthy dose will provide you with the building blocks you need.

Moreover, all leafy greens, especially the dark greens, are packed with minerals that your body needs to maintain proper functioning. This is important when you consider the fact that the building blocks for the body are contained in the 90+ nutrients that are needed for a healthy body. These nutrients are found across a variety of plants. So, if you have a predominantly meat-based diet, you might be missing out on some of the most important nutrients that the body needs in order to keep fit and healthy.

Boosting the Immune System When on the Plant-Based Eating Plan and Through Supplementation

This is a legitimate question that comes up during this discussion. The fact of the matter is that we should all consume a vitamin and mineral supplement regardless of the type of diet we follow. It just makes sense to do so since the body needs a host of nutrients in order to function efficiently. As a result, a supplement helps fill the gaps that nutrition leaves behind.

While it's always a good idea to double-check with your doctor before taking any supplements, you can basically pick the supplement of your choice. It's a good idea to consume one that has a wide range of vitamins and minerals. These components help the body recover and regenerate many of the parts that get worn down over time. In some cases, chronic exposure to stress leaves considerable effects behind. Consequently, combining your new plant-based eating plan with a solid multivitamin and multimineral pack can help you get back on track.

Moreover, supplementation is a good idea when you have a demanding lifestyle, be it a result of physical exercise or working long hours. Please bear in mind that being able to put in a great deal of nutrients in your body will help it fight off common illnesses such as colds and the flu, while giving your immune system a fighting chance against any nasty bugs that might come your way.

Overall Health and Wellbeing

Most folks who make the switch over to the plant-based eating plan, describe feeling much "lighter" within the first few days. The reason for this is that your body begins an automatic detox program. By stopping the consumption of meat and other processed foods, you are allowing your body to get rid of these potentially toxic foods.

As your body begins to detox, your immune system, digestive tract, and metabolism all begin to function at a more efficient rate. The end result is a much lighter body. By "lighter" we mean that you are not carrying out as much potentially harmful substances as compared to the past.

To put this point into specific relief. When you are intoxicated by the foods you eat, it's quite common to feel a "full" stomach and experience bloating. This is a clear-cut sign that your body is going through an inflammatory process.

Can you stop this from happening?

Absolutely!

But you must focus on cutting out as much as you can of the processed foods you are eating in addition to meat. In fact, you will find that some folks in the health and fitness community go on "meat fasts" for short periods of time. What happens during this time is that a person will forego meat and animal products for a specific amount of time, say, a week or so. During this time, the intention is to help the body detox. When this happens, the resources the body has allocated to digesting meat are now assigned to other functions.

For instance, digesting meat requires a great deal of water. So, when you are digesting large amounts of meat, your body needs to consume lots of water just to flush out the meat you have eaten. This can leave you dehydrated. Consequently, you'll feel like you got run over by a train. When you stop eating as much meat or cut it out altogether, your body can now assign the water you consume to keeping your body hydrated. This is why many folks report higher levels of energy as compare to the past.

Is It Worth the Sacrifice?

Some folks look at switching over to a plant-based eating plan like a sacrifice. They feel like they are giving up on their favorite foods in favor of a healthier eating approach. The fact of the matter is that making this switch, even if it's just temporary, makes all the sense in the world. When you make this shift, your body will automatically begin to make the necessary adjustments.

The reality is that the downside to the plant-based eating plan is all in your head. You may think you lack the willpower to do it. Truthfully, you have it in you. All you need to do make a commitment to improving your overall health and wellbeing. When you begin to see the results, you won't want to go back.

Chapter 2: The Basics Of A Plant-Based Diet

What Is A Plant-Based Diet?

Some people are doing it; some people are talking about it, but there is still a lot of confusion about what a whole plant-based diet actually entails. Since we split food into their macronutrients: sugars, proteins, and fats, most of us are uncertain about nutrition. What if we were able to put these macronutrients back together again in order to free your mind from confusion and stress? The secret here is simplicity.

Whole foods are foods that come from the earth unprocessed. Now, on a whole food plant-based diet, we eat some minimally processed foods like whole bread, whole wheat pasta, tofu, nondairy milk, and some nuts and seed butter. All of these are fine as long as they are handled to a minimum. So here are the different categories:

- Legumes (basically lentils and beans) of whole grains.

- Fruits and vegetables

- Nuts and seeds (including nut butter)

- Herbs and spices

All categories mentioned above constitute an entire diet based on plants. How to prepare them is where the fun comes in; how to season and cook them; and how to mix and match to give them great flavor and variety in your meals. So long as you regularly eat these foods, you will forever forget about sugars, protein, and fat.

Now, some may say, "Well, I can't eat soy," "I don't like tofu," and so on. Well, the beauty of an entire diet based on food plants is that if you don't like some food, like soy, in this case, you don't have to eat it. In a whole plant-based diet, it is not a necessary component. Instead of barley, you can get brown rice, quinoa instead of wheat; I'm sure you catch the drift right now. It really does not matter. Only find the right thing for you.

Just because you decided to adopt a plant-based diet lifestyle, that doesn't mean it's a healthy diet. Plant-based diets have a fair share of junk and other unhealthy foods, case in point, regular veggie pizza, and non-dairy ice cream consumption. Staying healthy requires you to eat healthy foods – even in a dietary setting, based on plants.

A few words that fly around are a similar eating style, but they're both distinct. That doesn't mean you're going to have to tag yourself to adhere to that way of eating; these words define various ways of eating to help you understand what types of food choices are in a particular class. This analysis can also help you understand how a diet based on a crop blends into the larger picture.

- Plant-based: This way of eating is based on berries, vegetables, rice, legumes, nuts, and seeds with few or no foods of animal origin. The plant-based diet is preferably a vegan diet with some versatility in the intermediate stages, with the intention of becoming 100% plant-based over time.

- Vegan: It describes someone who eats nothing from an animal, be it fish, fowl, rodents, or insects. Vegans refrain from animal meats as well as from other animal-made foods (such as milk and honey). They also often abstain from buying, wearing or using any kind of animal products (e.g., leather).

- Fruit: it represents a vegan diet consisting primarily of fruit.

- Raw vegan: This is an uncooked vegan diet that often includes dehydrated foods.

- Vegetarian: Sometimes, this plant-based diet includes milk and eggs.

- Flexitarian: This plant-based diet includes the occasional meat or fish consumption. I like to call it "a little bit of this and a little bit of that" — said, of course, without judgment!

Why You Need To Cut Back On Processed And Animal-Based Products

You've probably heard that fast food is bad for you over and over again. "Avoid preservatives; avoid processed foods;" but no one really gives you any real or solid information about why they should be avoided and why they are dangerous. So, let's break it down so you can fully understand why these guilty culprits should be stopped.

They have huge addictive properties

We have a strong tendency as humans to be addicted to certain foods, but the fact is that it is not our fault entirely. Practically all of the unhealthy foods we indulge in activate our dopamine neurotransmitter brains from time to time. It makes the brain feel "healthy," but this is for only a short time. This also creates a tendency toward addiction; that's why somebody will always find themselves going back to another candy bar – even if they don't really need it. Through cutting the stimulus entirely, you will stop all this.

They are loaded sugar and high fructose corn syrup

Processed and animal-based products are loaded with sugars and high fructose corn syrup with a nutritional value that is close to zero. More and more studies are now showing what many people have always suspected; that genetically modified foods cause inflammation of the gut, which in turn makes it more difficult for the body to absorb essential nutrients. The downside of your body, from muscle loss and brain fog to fat gain, cannot be stressed enough if you fail to properly absorb essential nutrients.

They are loaded with refined carbohydrates

Processed foods are loaded with refined carbs and products based on animals. Yes, it is a fact that carbs are needed in your body to provide energy to perform body functions. However, the refining of carbs eliminates the essential nutrients; it eliminates the whole grain component by refining whole grains. After refining, what you're left with is what's called "empty" carbs. By spiking blood sugar and insulin levels, these can have a negative impact on your metabolism.

They are loaded with artificial ingredients

Your body treats them as a foreign object when you consume artificial ingredients. They become an invader in essence. The body is not used to accept things like sucralose or artificial sweeteners. So, your body is doing the best it can. It triggers an immune response that reduces your resistance to disease, making you vulnerable. Otherwise, your body's focus and energy on protecting your immune system could be diverted elsewhere.

They contain components that cause a hyper reward sense in your body

What this means is that they contain components such as monosodium glutamate (MSG), high-fructose corn syrup components, and certain colors that can carve addictive properties. They are encouraging your body to receive a reward from it. For example, MSG is present in many prepackaged pastries. What this does is that to enjoy the taste, it stimulates your taste buds. Just by the way your brain communicates with your taste buds, it becomes psychological.

This reward-based system makes your body want more and more, putting you at a severe risk of over-consumption of calories. What about food from animals? The term "low quality" is often used to refer to plant proteins as they tend to have lower amounts of essential amino acids than animal proteins. What most people don't realize is that more essential amino acids can be harmful to their health. Now, let's discuss more on that.

Animal Protein Lacks Fiber

Most people end up displacing the plant protein they already had in their quest to load more animal protein. This is poor because, unlike plant protein, animal protein lacks fiber, antioxidants, and phytonutrients. Fiber deficiency in various communities and societies around the world is quite common. According to the Institute of Medicine, for instance, in the USA, the average adult absorbs only about 15 grams of fiber per day relative to the 38 grams required. Lack of adequate intake of dietary fiber is associated with increased risk of colon and breast cancer, as well as disease of Crohn, heart disease, and constipation.

Animal protein causes a spike in IGF-1

IGF-1 is the growth factor-1-like hormone insulin. It stimulates cell division and growth, which may sound good but also stimulates cancer cell growth. Therefore, higher blood levels of IGF-1 are associated with increased risk of cancer, malignancy, and proliferation.

Animal protein contains high levels of phosphorus

Animal protein causes phosphorus to increase. By secreting a hormone called fibroblast growth factor 23 (FGF23), our bodies normalize the high levels of phosphorus. FGF23 was also found to cause irregular heart muscle enlargement—a risk factor in extreme cases of heart failure and even death.

Instead, given all the issues, the "high quality" of animal protein's aspect might be more appropriately described as "high risk." Like caffeine, which you will feel withdrawal symptoms after you completely cut it off, processed foods can be cut off immediately. Maybe the one thing you're going to lose is the comfort of not having to prepare every meal from scratch.

Plant-Based Diet Vs. Vegan

Mistaking a vegan diet for a plant-based diet or vice versa is quite common for people. Okay, although there are parallels between both diets, they are not quite the same. So let's really break it down quickly.

Vegan

A vegan diet is one that does not include products based on animals. This includes meat, dairy, eggs, and products or ingredients such as honey derived from animals. Someone who describes himself as a vegan carries this perspective into their daily lives. What this means is that they are not using or encouraging the use of clothing, boots, accessories, shampoos, and make-up made from animal products. For example, wool, beeswax, leather, gelatin, silk, and lanolin are included. People's inspiration to live a vegan lifestyle also comes from an urge to stand up and fight animal mistreatment and bad animal ethical treatment, as well as to support animal rights.

Plant-Based Diet

On the other hand, an entire diet based on food plants shares a similarity with veganism in the sense that it does not also promote the dietary consumption of products based on animals. It covers eggs, meat, and dairy. What's more, unlike the vegan diet, the diet does not include processed foods, white flour, oils, and refined sugars. The aim here is to create a diet of unprocessed vegetables, herbs, whole grains, nuts, seeds and legumes that are minimally processed.

The health benefits it offers are often guided by full-food plant-based diet followers. It is a diet that has very little to do with calorie restriction or macro counting, but mostly with disease prevention and reversal.

Getting Started On A Whole Food

Plant-Based Diet

Common misconceptions among many people – even some in the health and fitness industry – is that anyone who switches to a plant-based diet becomes super healthy automatically. There are plenty of plant-based junk foods out there, such as non-dairy ice cream and frozen veggie pizza, which can really destroy your health goals if you consume them all the time. The only way you can achieve health benefits is to commit to healthy foods. On the other hand, in keeping you inspired, these plant-based snacks play a role. In moderation, sparingly and in small bits, they should be consumed. So, this is how you get started on a whole plant-based recipe without further ado.

Decide What a Plant-Based Diet Means for You

The first step is to make a decision to structure how your plant-based diet will look, and it will help you transition from your current dietary outlook. This is really personal, something that varies from person to person. While some people choose not to tolerate any animal products at all, some occasionally do with tiny bits of milk or meat. Deciding what and how you want your plant-based diet to look like is really up to you. The most important thing is that you must make a large majority of your diet from whole plant-based foods.

Understand What You Are Eating

Okay, now that you have taken the decision, your next step will require a great deal of analysis on your side. What do we mean by this? Well, if this is your first time trying out the plant-based diet, you may be surprised by the number of foods that contain animal products, especially packaged foods. When shopping, you'll find yourself cultivating the habit of reading tags. This points out that many pre-packaged foods contain animal products, and if you only want to stick to plant products for your new diet, you need to keep a close eye on the labeling of the ingredients. Maybe you've decided to allow a certain amount of animal products in your diet; well, you're just going to have to watch out for foods filled with oils, sugars, salt, preservatives, and other items that might have an effect on your healthy diet.

Find Revamped Versions of Your Favorite Recipes

I'm sure you've got a number of favorite, not necessarily plant-based dishes. Leaving everything behind is typically the hardest part for most people. There's still a way to meet you halfway, though. Take some time to talk about those non-plant-based foods that you like. Think along the lines of flavor, texture, versatility, and so on; and look for swaps in the entire diet based on food plants that can fulfill what you're missing.

Build a Support Network

It's hard to build a new habit, but it doesn't have to be. Find some friends, or even family members, who are happy to be with you in this lifestyle. This will help you stay focused and inspired while also having a form of transparency and emotional support. You can do fun things like trying out and sharing with these friends new recipes or even hitting up restaurants that offer a variety of plant-based choices. You can even go a step further and look up local social media plant-based groups to help you expand your network of knowledge and support.

Getting To The Root Of A Plant-Based Diet

You'll find so many interesting things to learn and try, but I'm bringing you to the basics for now and asking you which foods to avoid.

Valuable vegetables

You'll find a whole variety of vegetables that you'll really get to know quite well when eating plant-based veggies. If you're new to this, at the beginning, you're likely to stick to tried-and-true, popular veggies because they're going to feel healthy. These vegetables are a good start:

- Beets

- Carrots

- Kale

- Parsley, basil, and other herbs

- Spinach

- Squash

- Sweet potatoes

Fantastic fruits

We all love it! You need to get on this train if you haven't because the fruits are delicious; sweet; full of sugar, color, and beautiful vitamins; and so, so good for you.

- Apples

- Avocado

- Bananas

- Blueberries

- Coconut

- Mango

- Pears

- Pineapple

- Raspberries

- Strawberries

Wonderful whole grains

Consuming whole grains of good quality is a healthy part of a diet based on vegetables. Don't worry; you can still have your pastas and breads, but the key word here is "whole." You don't want the real thing to be polished or stored. When purchasing these items, make sure that the only ingredient is the grain itself. While it is possible to purchase proper whole grains in packaging from the shelf, make sure that you double-check the label to confirm that it is indeed a whole grain (and just a whole grain).

- Brown rice

- Brown-rice pasta

- Quinoa Rolled oats

- Sprouted-grain spelt bread

Lovable legumes

Learning to love beans on a plant-based diet is important because they are a great source of food, protein, and fuel. It may take you and your body a while to get used to them, but they will soon be your friends – especially when you find out how great it is to eat them in soups, salads, burgers, and other creative media. Here are some of the best things to begin with:

- Black beans

- Chickpeas

- Kidney beans

- Lentils

- Split peas

Notable nuts and seeds

A decent handful of nuts is good. But the thing about eating them on a plant-based diet is to make sure they're unsalted, unoiled, and raw. You can feel free to eat them in moderation alongside your other wonderful plant-based foods as long as you enjoy them in their natural state. Here are the best to begin with:

- Almonds

- Cashews

- Chia seeds

- Flaxseeds

- Hempseeds

- Pumpkin seeds

- Sunflower seeds

- Walnuts

Chapter 3: What You Stand To Gain From A Plant-Based Diet

Plants as a Medicine

Medicine has always been made using plants. It is therefore crystal clear that the plant-based diet can serve as medicines to our bodies.

You may find that when a person is unwell, a health expert may recommend eating a particular plant-based food. This is because plants have always had medicinal properties.

Diet-Related Diseases

Some of the diseases that are diet-related include;

Diabetes

Cancer

Cardiac arrest

Foods that Reduce Inflammation

If you already eat a fairly healthy diet, you will have no trouble incorporating these foods into your meals. In fact, you may already be enjoying them and just need a few tweaks to increase their presence in your meal planning. Some of the good foods that prevent and reduce chronic inflammation are as follows:

Omega 3 Fatty Acids

Omega 3 fatty acids are found in fish and fish oil. They calm the white blood cells and help them realize there is no danger, so they will return to dormancy.

Fruits And Vegetables

Most fruits and vegetables are anti-inflammatory. They are naturally rich in antioxidants, carotenoids, lycopene, and magnesium. Dark green leafy vegetables and colorful fruits and berries do much to inhibit white blood cell activity.

At least nine servings of fruits and vegetables each day are recommended. One serving is about a half-cup of cooked fruits and vegetables or a full cup if raw. The Mediterranean Diet, rich in fruits and vegetables, is often suggested to individuals suffering from chronic inflammation.

Protective Oils And Fats

Yes, there are a few oils and fats that are actually good for chronic inflammation sufferers. They include coconut oil and extra virgin olive oil.

Fiber

Fiber keeps waste moving through the body. Since the vast majority of our immune cells reside in the intestines, it is important to keep your gut happy. Eat at least 25 grams of fiber every day in the form of fresh vegetables, fruits, and whole grains. If that doesn't provide enough fiber, feel free to take a fiber supplement.

Flavor your food with spices and herbs instead of bad fats and unsafe oils. Spices like turmeric, cumin, cloves, ginger, and cinnamon can enhance the calming of white blood cells. Herbs like fennel, rosemary, sage, and thyme also aid in reducing inflammation while adding delicious new flavors to your food.

Healthy snacks would include a limited amount of unsweetened, plain yogurt with fruit mixed in, celery, carrots, pistachios, almonds, walnuts, and other fruits and vegetables.

Plants for Weight Loss

Obesity is considered to be an epidemic nowadays. Shockingly, more than 69 percent of adults in the United States are considered obese or overweight. Making changes in your diet and your whole lifestyle can lead to drastic weight loss when done properly. The impacts of these changes can be promising and long lasting. There are numerous studies that determined plant-based diet plans are very effective for weight loss.

The whole-food plant-based diet plan is rich in fiber and restricts processed foods while forbidding soda, refined grains, fast food, candy, and added sugars, making it ideal for weight loss. An overall assessment of 12 research studies found that people who followed plant-based diet plans lost more weight (2 kg less, in almost 18 weeks as compared to non-plant-based diet followers). Therefore a plant-based diet plan can also keep you from gaining weight.

You can eat:

- All vegetables, including greens like spinach, kale, chards, collards, asparagus, broccoli, cauliflower, bell peppers, tomatoes, onion, etc

- All fruits, including berries, avocado, apple, banana, watermelon, grapes, oranges, etc

- Plant-based alternates to meat like tofu and tempeh

- Plant-based milk and dairy products including coconut milk, almond milk, peanut butter, almond butter, cashew yogurt, etc

- All whole-grains, including brown rice, amaranth, quinoa, barley, all beans, whole wheat pasta, whole-grain bread, etc

- All nuts, including cashews, almonds, walnuts, macadamia nuts, etc

- All seeds like chia seeds, flaxseed, hempseeds, etc

- Lentils

- Millets

- Flax eggs

- Honey, maple syrup, coconut sugar, stevia, Splenda, erythritol, etc

- Unsweetened coffee and tea

You cannot eat:

- Meat including beef, pork, and poultry

- Seafood including fish and shrimps

- Processed animal products like hot dogs, sausages

- Dairy items like butter, eggs, whole milk, yogurt, etc

- Sweetened drinks like soda, fruit juices, sweetened tea and coffee

- Fried food and fast foods

- White bread and white pasta

Chapter 4: The Macro And Micro Essentials Of A Plant-Based Diet

A plant-based diet plan is a complete change of lifestyle, which is why it does not follow any strict rules for its configuration. You simply have to cut off animal-based foods entirely from your diet. Listed below are a few factors for a plant-based diet plan:

1. Eliminate animal-based foods.

2. Consume plants like seeds, legumes, fruits, veggies, nuts, and whole grains abundantly.

3. Emphasize more on the whole, natural, or minimally processed foods.

4. Eat locally-sourced and organic food when possible.

5. Cut off refined foods, including white flour, processed oils, and added sugars.

Most of the above traits are also found in vegetarian and vegan diet plans, which is why the whole-food plant-based diet is easily confused with them. But, trust us, they are different. A vegan diet eliminates all animal-related foods, including seafood, dairy, honey, meat, and poultry. On the other hand, vegetarian diets exclude meat and poultry but typically allow seafood, dairy products, eggs, and honey.

Contrary to them, the whole-food plant-based diet plan is more flexible and forgiving. The food is mostly plant-based, but you can also eat animal-based products in moderation. The extent of animal-related foods in your diet plan depends on your personal choice of entirely not eating them or consuming them in small amounts. In short, a whole-food plant-based diet plan is comprised of plant-based foods with a minimal amount of animal-related products and processed foods.

Plant foods possess most of the primary nutrients and their substituents, which are as follows: Protein Proteins are composed of amino acids, which are an essential source of energy in the human body. Quinoa contains all essential amino acids and is a rich source of proteins. Plants, such as nuts, beans, lentils, and soy seeds are a great source of proteins.

Vitamin B12

Vitamin B12 is abundantly acquired via fish, meat, dairy products, and eggs. However, a plant-based diet makes sure to make vitamin B12 available through fortified yeast, cereals, and soy milk. The deficiency of vitamin B12 causes anemia and nerve damage, so the followers of this diet can take supplements to avoid its lack.

Iron

The iron is an essential mineral that carries blood oxygen to different parts of the body. The plant food, which is an excellent source of iron, are dark green vegetables (spinach, kale, peas), whole grains, bread, nuts, seeds, dried beans, and cereals. The iron obtains from plant sources absorbs less as compared to the animal source. The absorption of plant-based iron can be increased with vitamin C.

Vitamin C

Vitamin C is vital for humans and oranges, kiwis, broccoli, strawberries, and tomatoes are good plant sources of vitamin C.

Vitamin D

Vitamin D is required for a healthy immune system, bones, and muscles. Plant sources of vitamin D are almond milk and some cereals.

Omega-3- Fatty acid

Omega 3 fatty acids play an essential role in reducing the risk of heart diseases and improving the immune system. Fatty fish and other seafood are the best sources for this nutrient. Omega 3 fatty acids can be obtained through various plant sources, including chia seeds, organic canola oil, flaxseeds, and flaxseed oil.

Zinc

Zinc is known to strengthen the immune system, assist wound healing, and maintaining blood sugar levels. Plant sources of zinc include tofu, whole grains, peas, tempeh, nuts, and lentils. Phyllates is a compound in plants that inhibits the absorption of zinc, so it is best to soak plants overnight.

Calcium

Bones and teeth are composed mainly of calcium. Calcium also improves nerves, muscles, and heart. Soy milk, almond, tofu, kale, bok choy, and broccoli are the best sources of calcium.

The first important tip is to get rid of meaty thoughts and personalize your plant-based diet plan by customizing your favorite recipes into this diet. You must try some new recipes with a different style for breakfast, lunch, dinner, snacks, and beverages. Your aim should be to stay as healthy as you could by abstaining from meat and dairy.

Macronutrients

Macronutrients are present in our diets at all times. Yet, tend to mix up the ratios somewhat, thereby leading to weight gain and an unhealthy balance in our diet. The main thing to keep in mind that there is no significant alteration between the plant-based eating plan and a regular meat-based diet. The important thing is to maintain that healthy ratio so that you can enjoy the largest amount of benefits.

In general, there are three large macronutrients: carbs, fats and protein. These three elements comprise the types of foods that you need to consume in order to lose weight and help your body improve its overall functioning.

Regularly, we tend to load up on carbs, have an increased fat intake and consume protein in relatively small quantities. This type of configuration makes it hard for your body to get the necessary nutrients to ensure proper health. On top of that, if you don't ensure that you're consuming enough fruits and vegetables, your body may be undernourished.

Now, some folks try to skirt the issue by taking a vitamin supplement, or even multiple supplements. That strategy may help reduce the gap, but it won't truly address the issue.

Think about it.

If you have a high-carb, low protein diet, no matter how many supplements you take, your body still has to deal with a large number of carbs. Therefore, you may not see the weight loss results you expect. So, that is why you need to think about how you can reduce your consumption of carbs (particularly refined carbs) and increase your intake of healthy fats and proteins.

For starters, a good rule of thumb is to adhere to the following ratio: 45% carbs, 35% fats and 20% protein. This ratio allows the body to consume enough carbs (after all, carbs are transformed into energy by the body) to fuel your day, enough fats, to allow bodily processes to function regularly such as hormone production and protein to enable muscle growth, cell repair and boost your immune system. With the plant-based eating plan, you can easily follow this ratio without having to wrack your brain trying to figure out where you can get this type of nutrients. Moreover, by reducing the number of carbs you consume, you can allow your body to begin tapping into its reserves. The reasoning behind this assumption lies in the fact that the body cannot continue to fuel its functions without fat. Since fat is transformed into energy, the body needs to take the fat that is being consumed and use it up. However, if the calories that are being consume are insufficient, then the body needs to make up the difference from its reserves. This is where weight loss happens. So, don't neglect your macronutrient groups. Foods like avocados and olive oil are a great source of healthy fats while nuts, beans and dark greens are great sources of protein. As for carbs, grains and cereals will get the job done.

Micronutrients

Micronutrients are just as important as macronutrients. They make up the specific elements that the body needs to function properly. These are the vitamins and minerals that the body requires in order to power the various operations it runs. In general, micronutrients are present in all of the foods that we consume. Of course, some have a larger concentration of these nutrients that others. Sadly, some have little to none of these elements. This is the reason why we keep underscoring the point about avoiding processed foods.

On the whole, processed foods have very little micronutrients present as they are generally eliminated during the processing portion. Processes such as bleaching, starching and so on eliminate most of the nutrients that the original source food has. These nutrients are replaced by salts and sugars which make these processed foodstuffs highly addictive.

In addition, meat lacks most of the micronutrients that are needed by the body as these nutrients are not always present in the muscle (meat is mainly muscle). Hence, meat is a great source of protein, but neglects to address the vast number of micronutrients that the body needs.

Examples of micronutrients include iron, magnesium, cobalt, selenium, copper, iodine and zinc, among many others. As for vitamins, these are A, C, D, the B group vitamins, in addition to others such as K which is used to promote healthy blood clotting (this is a major issue for diabetics in particular). Micronutrients are fundamental to a healthy body as they assist with specific functions throughout the body. A well-known example is vitamin C. Vitamin C is known to boost the immune system by allowing it to fuel cell repair. Furthermore, vitamin C is often prescribed as a cold remedy as it also strengthens the body's ability to fight off infection.

The most important thing to keep in mind is that all of the micronutrients are present in the various plants that we eat. Some have a higher concentration than others, while others may contain different elements as compared to others. This is why it is important to have a varied consumption of plants; in doing so, you can offer your body the various micronutrients it needs.

As always, a supplement can help bridge the gap. Supplementation can be part of your overall strategy, but it shouldn't be your excuse to cut out plants from your diet altogether.

Chapter 5: How To Eliminate Bad Eating Habits

Cooking is all about preparing food that best suits you with the rest of the family. We all cook food for different reasons or rather goals. Some objectives are good, while others might sound vague, but all in all, we all cook with one primary purpose of improving our health. We all try our best to make different plans for doing our kitchen work. It also becomes vital to make sure that everything comes out in its perfect order with enough tastes and flavors. Sometimes we go for taste and forget that the nutrients content also matters a lot, especially when our health is considered.

Our health has been a significant factor in many situations. Therefore, that's why we prefer to deal with anything affecting it, by all means, using different ways. We are more inclined to health issues when types of food we are preparing have been put into significant consideration. These types of food referred to junk foods, and most of them have got a higher level of meat as a single ingredient. They are preferred due to their quick or natural mode of preparation.

In many cases, this occurs without knowing that some food such as meat, if not well cooked, will accelerate the thriving conditions of the internal worms. These warms include tapeworms that have severe complications with the internal body organs. These people have beliefs that the best restaurants within the world have been reserved for some high-class personality. This is just a belief since anyone with enough resources can visit those high-end restaurants. But these restaurants are served meat-related foods that have severe complications within the long run. Even though we are much aware of this, many argue that they lack time to prepare plant-based meals. That being creative enough to play with the plant-based recipes are time-consuming.

This has eventually affected the lives of many. Many have got health issues that hinder them from being productive in their capacity or even at work. These health issues include cancer-related complications, especially within the colon, breast, and even prostate cancer. Obesity has been another health issue over the years now. Many studies have been

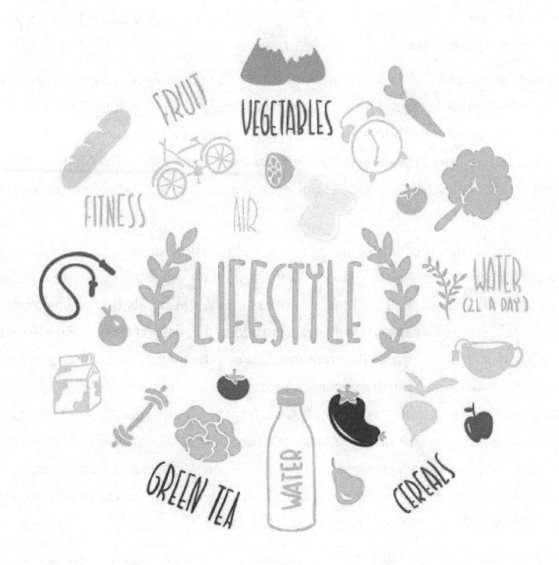

carried out on the possible ways to control these health issues, and many findings have narrowed down to plant-based cooking.

It is, therefore, possible for all of us to look for critical ways to understand plant-based food and how we can embark on it. Understanding plant-based cooking will even make you better and start making or preparing excellent plant-based meals, which are delicious and yummy. This knowledge will also help you in indulging in this kind of diet that you have never belonged to. Over some time, your cooking skills will improve, and having these basics; you will never require additional time or effort to prepare this food. You will be ultimately an experienced guru in the field of cooking plant-based meals without following even the recipes.

The plant-based cooking or preparation of food can be precisely defined as the type of cooking which involves or revolves around food prepared from plants. This implies that your diet will have more plant food as compared to other kinds of food. In other words, your food will be more of plant sources than meat and sometimes will even have no traces of meat at all — these diets composed of nuts, legumes, beans, whole grains and much more.

Apart from that, the nutrition recommendation also covers almost all types of vitamins. These meals have higher levels of fiber. They also contain other types of nutrients needed within the body. This type of cooking also offers enough minerals that are helpful in the optimal healthy life of a person, thus leading to a long lifespan. They also and also act as a preventive mechanism towards different diseases or infections. These diseases arise from heart complications and involve coronary thrombosis and other blood-related disorders such as blockage of blood vessels and much more. These types of food comprise of vegetables and fruits which have red, orange and yellow colors such as carrots, tomatoes, mangoes and much more. The same also includes green vegetables such as spinach, kales, romaine lettuce, broccoli, bok choy, among others. Traces of leeks, onions and even garlic can also be regarded as part and parcel of phytonutrient.

Plant-based cooking has more to offer in terms of disease curbing. As usual, this is compared to a vegetarian diet. The same meal plan is also compared to the Mediterranean diet even though the latter two have been found to support the health issues. This also leads us to an urge to understand these differences to be able to comprehensively understand what we shall be doing in the kitchen when preparing plant-based dishes.

The Mediterranean diet has its initial roots from plant-based sources and also incorporates other foods like fish, yogurt, poultry, and so on. Things such as meat and sweets are offered in fewer quantities even though not very often. This Mediterranean diet has been inclined to the positive side of our health. Studies have shown that the risk of getting heart diseases have reduced tremendously. There is a decreased level of metabolic syndrome with a good number of people showing a reduction in the level of health issues arising from this syndrome. Cases like cancers have also reduced.

This diet was found to be of help to people suffering from cancerous diseases such as colon, prostate, and even breast cancer. With this diet, if well offered, the frailty in older people will reduce too. This diet can also help to improve the functionality of your brain and physical body in general. However, this diet is slightly different from a vegetarian diet.

A vegetarian diet is gotten purely from plant-based meals. The same meal is also harvested from cooking meals with the plan in mind. Currently, only a few people are taking additional dietary supplements.

Vitamin B12 is one of these supplements. It's used to help their consumers in acquiring all the nutrients needed by their bodies. The vegetarian diets come in handy in different forms or rather types. It's now upon you to choose the best that fits you and the rest of your family. It is good to understand that your health issues should give you a direction when it comes to choosing the type of vegetarian food. There are different types which include a semi-vegetarian diet. This type consists of eggs, products of dairy, meat but not always, seafood, fish, and even poultry. A different kind of vegetarian diet is a pescatarian. It also includes eggs, it has fish in it, has seafood and some dairy products. However, this diet lacks meat or poultry. The last type though not often is called lactose vegetarian diet, which comprises using eggs and dairy foods only. This implies that this diet does not entertain anything to do with meat, fish, poultry, or even seafood.

Another related plant-based diet is the Nordic diet. This diet has some features similar to the Mediterranean cooking plan. It also has a high level of whole grains and berries. Other meals that you can look at include fatty fish such as salmon and so on. There are also vegetables, fruits, and even legumes. This diet also contains eggs and some dairy products with a high limitation of red meat and other processed foods. It does not involve sweets too.

The human race is funny when it comes to choosing between a diet comprising of meat in abundance supply and the one which has plant-based sources. It is now clear that many people eat meat not because of its nutritional value but because of its taste. They have forgotten that flavor and nutrition cannot go hand in hand. They are always going into different directions. The same implies that it will take some more time to instill this kind of information into the current generation. For them to digest it, they will still need much more time. And as a result of this, many will suffer from health-related diseases.

Many people argue that the actual plant-based cooking plan has no dairy and its products, that they have no meat at all or even oils and eggs. Many seem not to understand the difference that has been stipulated above concerning vegetarian diets, Mediterranean food, and even Nordic dishes. Others go ahead to hardening of the blood vessels such as arteries which later lead to heart disease.

Again there are a lot of talks that cover the consumption of eggs and meat. In the opinion of such individuals, the incorporation and their intake lead to the thriving of cancerous cell multiplication. It's now clear that many people have had a severe misconception about foods like oils. Surprisingly, to some point, they are not aware of the sources of these oils to be from plants like sunflower, avocados, canola, or even olives.

We are much obsessed with the word "plant" without taking much consideration, the word "plant-based." And, in this scenario, many argue that dairy products even if offered in fewer quantities, will still have various side effects on the body. This is true based on the knowledge that these fewer quantities are critical supplements in the building of muscles. Apart from that, the meals also lower blood pressure. This low quantity also helps in the reduction of tooth decay, reduces obesity, and also can help in the prevention of cancer.

Many people have argued that diet is perfect for your health. However, when it comes to discussing some of the issues affecting our bodies, the results have been overwhelming towards the plant-based meals. The idea is based on the fact that it can quickly help in curbing and controlling many diseases.

A group of scholars, however, argued that, even though plant-based meal plans are best for our diets, not all should be preferred. Their study found that the best plant-based meal plans are those who emphasized on ingredients that are fresh and whole. And due to this, they cautioned on the use of processed plant foods like fully refined maize flour, fully refined wheat flour and so on. As a result, they argued that when all these are observed, then the issue of health will be solved a notch higher. All these are meant to help us understand the plant-based cooking and their benefits. Understanding the plant-based diet plan can be a cumbersome task, especially when you have a family who hates fruits and vegetables. The only way to go about it is to show them the source of food.

It's also vital to discuss the side effects of the food on the body. Besides, it's essential to provide good reasons why the best options for cooking are embracing organic meals and natural cooking meals. Giving a clear view on why some foods are better than others will at least help them to understand the plant-based cooking. Also, having that passion and love boosts the morale of adopting plant-based sources of food.

The first benefit of understanding plant-based cooking is that it will help us in restoring our health and curbing of diseases. Many studies have proved beyond doubts that focussing on the plant-based cooking plan helps a lot in returning our healthy initial condition or rather situation. This involves the entire use of these meals in our daily diets. Diseases like cancer, especially cancer of the colon, prostate cancer, and even breast cancer, have been found to have a negative result with the plant-based foods. This implies that the cancerous cells are entirely affected by the presence of this food within the body system. As a result, their day to day thriving or growing is diminished and may even fail to show up. Due to this, the effect of cancer reduces, and those already diagnosed can also get healed.

Again, people who are mainly into this diet are not risky in cases or issues touching disease. Therefore they will never be prone to this disease. Following this diet will tremendously reduce heart-related conditions such as coronary thrombosis, arteriosclerosis, and so on. This leads to enough flow of blood within the blood vessels and with the required pressure. As a result, cases of heart attack will be nothing to worry about. We have other kinds of blood-related diseases such as elephantiasis which come as a result of poor blood circulation within the lower organs of the body, especially the limbs. Well, observation and considering this diet will help us to eliminate this.

Understanding of plant-based food or meal plans can also help us in improving our way of eating. The idea refers to eating habits. We are coming from a rigid society obsessed with much technology that doesn't allow us to concentrate on plant-based food. This over obsession, especially on fast food such as junks and the rest, has misled us to channel our way to poor eating habits.

With the help of this handbook, we can improve our eating habits. With that said, excellent plant-based meal plans have an accurate idea of what to eat and when to it. The same implies that the meal has specified breakfast, lunch as well as supper. At the same time, snacks and dinner have been organized categorically.

We are living in a world where taste seems to be better than nutrition. A good number of people eat junk foods, especially meat just because of how these food taste and not their value. This leads to a high level of build-up fats within the muscles and walls of the stomach. Unhealthy eating habits later result in obesity and other health-related diseases. By understanding the benefits of plant-based cooking, we get the chance to meet a world free from excess unhealthy meals such as junk food. The case also implies that the level of meat-related disease is reduced. Plant-based diets eliminate all these thus making us lead a good and a better life.

Our understanding of plant-based food or rather meal plans help us to decrease in weight. That's losing weight. Plant-based cooking relies mainly on foods that have their sources from plants. These types of foods include vegetables like kales, spinach, broccoli, and much more. This diet also contains fruits like mangoes, tomatoes, lettuce, and so forth. Cereals such as wheat, maize flour, oats, and much more are also part of this.

When plant-based cooking plans are fully understood and followed, health sectors within the society or a community improves. Lots of medications become a past tense thing. The people live a happy life. The immune system of everyone increases and falling sick diminishes. As a result, drugs become eliminated or somewhat reduced to a minimal level. The same instance will lead to a rise in the economy within the community since not much will be spent on medication. This is made possible by the help of a careful comprehension of plant-based cooking. An excellent plant-based diet also has fewer complications within the body as compared to the diets full of meat and other fatty foods. And due to this, there is no build-up of disease within the body tissues that will eventually require medications.

Knowledge of plant-based cooking if fully implemented can help us eradicate cruelty within the world, thus making the sustainability of the world to be more manageable. Chaos and cruelty always come as a result of sheer misunderstanding within different sectors. This is the same for even health sectors. Maintaining good health is the main objective of our daily lives, and without doing this, then the world will be full of chaos.

Imagine a world where the health sector is below standards. This implies that many people will be suffering from diseases such as heart attacks plus other blood related or heart-related diseases. This will eventually leave many industries with fewer people in terms of employees. Competent personnel within the ranks of the company will reduce, and obesity increases. All these will create cruelty and chaos that will be hard to eradicate. In a situation where the knowledge of this diet is well understood, then the correct implementation is followed, chances of cruelty become low. This makes the world to be easily manageable.

This type of diet always saves time. Also, its preparation is based on cooking using the purest forms of recipes. The result is you enjoying a healthy diet. Additional cooking and meal preparation plans don't involve complicated methods that take time to understand. All the skills required to make these recipes are easy to acquire. The duration of cooking is also less since they take the shortest time possible to get prepared. This leads to saving of your precious time that can be invested in other productive responsibility within the community or in an organization. Understanding the plant-based cooking diet will eventually allow us to be more productive in other areas since preparations of these foods require less time.

These types of food from plant-based sources require less fuel. A less or little amount of energy will often be used in their preparations. As a result, energy is saved. When this occurs, the high energy levels lead to a better economy. The world economies grow and thrive well. A good economy is characterized by good governance. Apart from that, the people comprising that economy will lead a better life. The result is usually courtesy of our well comprehensive nature towards our plant-based cooking.

Chapter 6: Planning And Stocking Your Pantry

Unlike with other diet programs, with the plant-based diet, you don't have to worry too much about getting stared.

As you will find out for yourself, getting started is not that difficult because most likely, you are already eating most of what is required. There's a big chance that you will only need to make minimal changes in your diet.

Here are the steps on how to get started:

Step # 1 – Write down your current diet Do not make any changes with your diet first. For the first week, record all the dishes and snacks that you eat throughout the day. This will show you what areas in your food habits are necessary to be changed, and which ones can be retained.

Step # 2 – Write down a menu based on this diet Once you're done with recording the past week's diet, you can now create your diet for the second week. Take note that you don't have to completely overhaul your diet immediately as this will make the transition too drastic and might not provide positive results.

Start avoiding some of the foods and drinks that are not encouraged in a plant-based diet. You should also start adding more fruits and vegetables to dishes that you love. For example, if you are fond of eating oatmeal in the morning, it would be a great idea to start packing it with bananas, apples and mangoes. If you love snacking on yogurt, make it a point to stir in some blueberries or strawberries.

Step # 3 – Cut down on meat consumption Do not completely avoid all types of meat. But you just have to reduce intake slowly but surely. For instance, instead of eating steak with mashed potatoes on the side for dinner, why don't you try sautéing green beans with a few strips of beef and serve it with mashed potatoes on the side. This way, there are more vegetables than meat in your dish.

Step # 4 – Fill your pantry with healthy items It's a lot harder to adopt a healthy diet if you kitchen is filled with all sorts of junk foods. Discard the candies, sweet treats, sugary beverages and bags of chips that are in your pantry. Replace these with natural and healthy snacks like kale chips, whole grain bread slices, and fruit desserts.

What to Eat

Here's a list of all the foods and drinks that you should focus on while on a plant-based diet:

- ✓ Fruits – Apples, bananas, blueberries, blackberries, pears, oranges, mangoes, avocados, pineapple, strawberries, raspberries

- ✓ Vegetables – Spinach, tomatoes, carrots, cucumber, zucchini, potatoes, squash, broccoli, cauliflower, kale, cabbage

- ✓ Whole grains – Brown rice, quinoa, oats, barley, whole wheat bread, whole wheat pasta

- ✓ Legumes – Peanuts, beans, peas, chickpeas, lentils

- ✓ Plant-based protein – Tempeh, tofu

- ✓ Nuts – Almonds, walnuts, pistachios

- ✓ Nut butters

- ✓ Seeds – Sunflower seeds, flax seeds

- ✓ Healthy oils – Olive oil, avocado oil, grapeseed oil

- ✓ Herbs and spices

- ✓ Water

- ✓ Coffee

- ✓ Tea

- ✓ Smoothies

- ✓ Fresh fruit or veggie juices

Now, here's a list of all the foods and drinks that you can consume but try to limit intake as much as possible.

- Meat – Beef, pork, lamb

- Poultry – Chicken, turkey

- Seafood – Fish, shells, crabs, shrimp

- Dairy products – Milk, cheese, yogurt

- Processed meats - Bacon, sausage

What to Avoid

This one is a list of the foods and drinks that you would want to avoid as much as possible.

- Fast food

- Sweetened beverages

- Refined grains – White bread, white rice, refined pasta

- Packaged foods – Cookies, chips, cereals

TIPS

Make the transition for you easier using the following tips and strategies:

Make a meal planner

Write down a menu for the week or for the month so you don't have to worry about steering away from your healthy diet. It would be a good idea to make use of an online meal planner that you can access even when you're outside your home. But if you prefer to do it the traditional way, and write it on paper, that is a good idea too.

Eat small healthy snacks during the day

Doing this will keep you full longer and will reduce the possibility of getting tempted to eat foods that are not encouraged in a plant-based diet. If you are full, there's less tendency for you to crave for a huge slab of steak for instance.

Don't be too hard on yourself

Making a transition from one diet to another is always difficult and challenging. Do not expect yourself to be immediately comfortable with your new diet. It may take you longer than a week. It would probably require you at least a month to ease in to your new diet, even if this is not as restrictive as other types of diet.

Use meat as garnish

Instead of making it the centerpiece of your dish, use it as an "add-on". Instead of serving steak with a small amount of steamed veggies on the side, it would be better to turn things around and serve more steamed veggies and just a little amount of meat.

Use good fats

Make it a point to use only healthy fats like olive oil, avocados, nut butter and so on.

Have lots of salads

Salads are a great way to turn your regular diet into one that's plant-based. Not only that, these are extremely convenient to prepare and will only take you a few minutes to prepare. You won't have to spend a long time in the kitchen to cook an elaborate meal.

Satisfy cravings for sweets with fruits

There will always be those times when you will crave for something sweet. For some people, this usually happens after a meal. Do not deprive yourself. Instead, satisfy your craving the healthy way—eat fruits for dessert.

Follow these tips to ensure to have a smooth transition from your old diet into this new one. It may not be as challenging as with other diet programs, but of course, there will also be certain drawbacks that you would want to be prepared for.

Basic Shopping List

Shopping for a plant-based diet plan sounds tough, but it is pretty much easier. We are providing you with a list of foods that you can opt for while following the diet plan. You don't need to stick solely to this list; rather we recommend making changes to make the diet plan more versatile. The only thing to keep in mind is that it should be having plant-based ingredients. One more important thing to understand is that the formulation of products might change, so you have to keep a close eye on the labels on foods. The list includes the following:

1.   Fresh Produce (Veggies and Fruits) You can have a wide variety of fresh vegetables and fruits. Go for various dark leafy green veggies. We recommend avoiding avocados if you have cardiac complications and eat more if you are aiming to lose weight.

2.   Legumes and Beans You can enjoy all variants of lentils and dried beans. In case you opt for canned beans, prefer going for no salt or low-sodium. If you are unable to find any no-salt-added beans, rinse the beans thoroughly before using them.

3.   Seeds, Nuts, and Dried Fruits Don't go for nuts if you have cardiac complications and eat more of them if you wish to lose weight. In case you opt for nuts, every variant is better but prefer going for no-oil added or raw. Don't eat them by the handful as their fat content is high, and so is their calorie content, and it can make you overeat it. You can also use nut butter.

You can go for omega-3 rich flax and chia seeds for topping cereals and even replacing eggs in your baking recipes. The content should be 1 tbsp. of chia or ground flaxseed in addition to 3 tbsp of water, which is the equivalent of 1 egg. Whole flax seeds are hard to digest, so prefer going for ground flaxseed, or you can grind them in a coffee grinder before usage. Eat more seeds like pumpkin seeds, sesame, and sunflower seeds, etc.

Go for dried fruits, but keep in mind that they are not having any added sugar. One more important thing to remember is that that are having higher calories than fresh fruits. If you have a diabetic condition or are aiming to lose weight, prefer going for fresh fruits instead of dried ones. Moreover, avoid having dried banana chips as they are fried most of the time.

4.   Frozen Fruits You can have all types of frozen veggies and fruits without having

dairy ingredients or added oil.

You can also have a wide variety of whole-grain rice like long, medium, and short-grain, black, red, purple, wild, jasmine, and much more. You can have any type of rice, but not white rice on the plant-based diet plan.

You can have a wide array of whole-grain flours in your diet plan too. These include:

- Whole wheat pastry flour
- White whole wheat flour
- Whole wheat flour
- Oat Flour
- Barley Flour
- Amaranth Flour
- Rye Flour
- Spelt Flour
- Kamut Flour

Apart from these, you can also go for gluten-free flours if you are having any allergies to wheat. But it is important to read the labels carefully as various gluten-free flours are processed.

Mustards: You are not allowed to have high sugar honey mustard sauces.

Capers: You should rinse it before usage for minimizing the sodium content.

Olives: Go for olives that are not packed in oil, sparingly use them as they are very high in sodium.

Cheese Substitutes You should go for nutritional yeast for sprinkling purposes on pasta and even use it in recipes for adding a "cheesy" flavor to them. Special occasion's option includes: • Miyoko's Creamery cheeses (choose the no added oil varieties) • Miyoko's

Creamery cheeses (choose the no added oil varieties) They are very high in fat, so you have to use them in a moderate manner.

Chapter 7: Plant-Based Foods That Boost Your Immunity

Kiwis

Can reduce the length of the common cold. Can also help reduce the risk of children getting sick. Kiwis have high levels of vitamin C, antioxidants, folate, and potassium. The whole fruit can be eaten, including the peel, which can triple the amount of fiber. The peel also contains a special prebiotic that can be highly beneficial to microbiomes. A study reviewed in the Canadian Journal of Physiology revealed how green and gold kiwi fruits can help improve immune functioning and even provide extra protection against the cold and flu (Stonehouse, Gammon, Beck, Conlon, Von Hurst, & Kruger, 2013). This study showed that since kiwi are high in vitamin C, E, and K as well as antioxidants that those in higher risk groups, such as children and older adults, consuming this fruit can help give extra support to the immune system to fight off infections will also reduce the severity of symptoms.

Blueberries and other berries

Berries contain vitamin C antioxidants that prevent inflammation and cell damage. They provide the body with a chemical known as anthocyanins, that can help prevent colds, urinary tract infections, and reduce high blood pressure. Blueberries contain a high amount of pterostilbene which helps boost the immune system naturally. A case study published in Molecular Nutrition and Food Research analyzed the compounds to boost immunity and found that the most impactful was pterostilbene (Robbins, 2018). Berries are a great addition to salads, oatmeal, and muffins or pancakes.

Broccoli and other Cruciferous Vegetables

A study performed on mice, led by Dr. Stockinger, showed that mice who ate cruciferous vegetables were able to better fight off intestinal pathogens ("Cruciferous vegetables help," 2017). Cruciferous vegetables are necessary for optimal immune system functioning. This includes foods like kale, collard greens, mustard greens, bok choy, broccoli, and brussels sprouts. Kale provides you with the most beneficial anti-inflammatory agents. They contain beta-carotene, vitamin C, E, and K, folate, lutein, and zeaxanthin. They also provide you with sulfur substances, glucosinolates, which makes a phytochemical that boosts the immune system and produces anti-cancer agents.

Ginger

Ginger is a powerful anti-inflammatory and antioxidant, that contains antimicrobial properties to defend against infectious diseases. Gingerol, found in ginger, gives it its anti-cancer properties. Ginger root can be easily found and stored in the freezer. There are also dried, powdered, and oil forms of ginger.

Green Tea

One of the most powerful teas around. It contains catechins, antioxidants, quercetin, and L-theanine, all of which effectively fight off viruses and infections (Robins, n.d.). It has even been shown that drinking green tea regularly can help reduce the risk of cancers (Robins, n.d.).

Aside from the foods mentioned above you should aim to include these superfoods into your diet as well.

- Matcha
- Kale
- Spinach
- Goji berries
- Elderberries
- Chia seeds

- Sunflower seeds
- Pumpkin seeds
- Yogurt
- Bell peppers
- Turmeric
- Cinnamon

- Almonds
- Citrus fruits
- Mushrooms
- Chickpeas
- Salmon
- Sardine

Foods That Hinder the Immune System

Fast foods aren't just bad for your waistline but eating greasy foods from most chain fast food places can negatively impact your health. This is because these foods, which are often high in sugar and low in fiber, which can reprogram the response of the immune system. Continually consuming these foods puts the immune system in high alert and it responds as though there is a constant threat. This constant high alert puts unnecessary stress on the immune system. And even when you switch to eating a healthier diet, and eliminate fast food, the immune system still stays on high alert which can cause negative health problems (Allen, n.d.).

Monosodium glutamate (MSG) can cause oxidative stress to the spleen and thymus, which affects lymphocytes, whose job is to remove foreign invaders from the body and to produce antibodies. The lymphocytes produced are typically fewer and function improperly, which can trigger an immune overreaction. Removing MSG from your diet can help reverse the negative effects over time (Allen, n.d.).

Alcohol reduces the function of macrophages, the cells that attack foreign invaders, throws off immunoglobulin and cytokine levels, can impair the production of T and B-cells, as well as disrupt Circadian rhythm or sleep cycles (Allen, n.d.).

Caffeine can boost cortisol levels which is a hormone released when feeling stressed. This can affect your mood and metabolism. T-cell production can also be reduced when consuming caffeine regularly, resulting in your lymphocytes being suppressed and interleukin production to lower (Allen, n.d.).

Aside from the foods mentioned above you should avoid these foods as much as possible.

- Coffee
- Energy drinks
- Diet Pop/Soda
- Fried foods
- Fast foods
- MSG food
- Alcohol
- Fruits and vegetables treated with pesticides
- Processed sugar
- Refined oils
- Additives
- Processed flour or Gluten

Foods to Avoid with an Autoimmune Disease

Those with an autoimmune disease can be more sensitive to certain foods. These foods can also worsen symptoms and can make the condition worsen at a more progressive rate. Those with an autoimmune disease will often follow a strict autoimmune diet which focuses on eating primarily fresh fruits and vegetables, as well as healthy fats and fish.

Foods that should be avoided when you have an autoimmune disease include:

- Caffeine
- Alcohol

- Sugar

- Grains

- Dairy

- Red meat

Artificial Sweeteners

Many people look for a sugar substitute to replace the everyday white processed sugar found in many homes. Artificial sweeteners are often thought to be better for your health, but they are synthetic sweeteners that are primarily made from chemicals and all-natural sources are processed out.

The most common artificial sweeteners are:

- Saccharin

- Aspartame

- Acesulfame potassium or Ace-K

- Sucralose

- Neotame

These are often considered a great alternative because most contain no calories and are used in a number of packages that claim to have "no sugar added." Artificial sweeteners have been linked to a number of health issues such as obesity (Casey, Obert, Pearlman, 2017) . This is primarily due to artificial sweeteners interfering with signals in the body. The way the brain responds to these sweeteners also changes. Because these sweeteners are not actually sugar, they also interfere with blood sugar levels and puts individuals at a higher risk for glucose intolerance (Chodosh,2018).

Environmental Risks

It was thought that genes and age often determined who was susceptible to a disease more, but now it is believed that the environment has a bigger impact. Environmental factors such as dust and air pollutants can trigger someone already at higher risk for disease to become ill. Respiratory infections are becoming prominent, resulting in death across the globe.

When babies and young children are exposed to these harmful environmental factors early in life, they become less resistant to diseases. Early exposure to air pollutants like cigarette smoke, pesticides, and pollution disrupt the proper development and functioning of the immune system. This can cause the immune system to be unable to identify harmful pathogens that enter the body or cause it to over-react to pathogens that should be considered harmless. While symptoms may not be present in the first years of life, many individuals who are exposed early on to harmful chemicals and toxins in their environment are more likely to develop cancer or other immune deficiencies.

How can you help reduce the risk of environmental factors on your immune system?

1. Avoid using products that contain harmful chemicals in your homes. Instead use baking soda and vinegar as a daily cleaner which is just as effective yet, less harmful.

2. Keep all heating and cooling ducts clean. Dust particles can stay in vents and turn into airborne irritants. Performing a yearly cleaning on your home's vents can reduce the number of irritants in your home.

3. Use air filters to remove irritants and pollutants from your home. You can also add air purifying plants to your home such as aloe vera, peace lily, spider plant, boston fern, or areca palms.

4. Using a water filtration or purifying system can also help reduce the risk of bacteria or harmful toxins that may be in your water systems.

Now that you have a better understanding of what vitamins, nutrients, and minerals your body needs, you might be wondering if you can get all you need just through your diet?

Chapter 8: Ten Plant-Based Beauty Treatments To Use On Your Skin Recipes

Avocado

Using avocado is an excellent, natural way to nourish and care

for your body without any abrasive chemicals. Essential and extra-virgin avocado oil has long been used in beauty products such as hair conditioners, moisturizers, cleansers, and facials.

This is because avocado is a rich source of several essential nutrients that refresh and moisturize your skin.

Scoop out the flesh of a ripe avocado, mash it in a bowl, and smear it on your skin for a nourishing mask. Leave it on for at least 20 minutes before washing it off.

Coconut

Coconut oil, which you can buy in glass bottles, makes a great moisturizer from head to toe, particularly for dry lips and rough hands and feet. You can even use it on your scalp and for your hair.

Raw Honey

Raw honey is incredible for your skin, thanks to its antibacterial properties and hefty serving of skin-saving antioxidants.

Whether you're looking for an inexpensive DIY solution or a powerful skin treatment, raw honey can help you regain your glow.

The best way to use honey is to apply it topically as is (undiluted). That way, your skin can

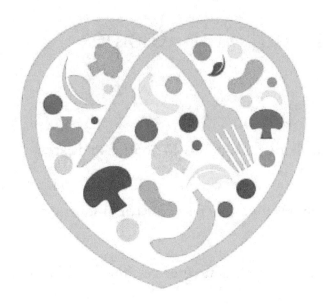

soak up all of its goodness.

After about 15 minutes, rinse it off. You may need two rinses to get it all off!

Lemon Juice

Fresh lemon juice has many benefits when applied directly to the skin.

The acids in lemon juice may be irritating to some people, so be sure to dilute lemon juice with water before applying it to your skin:

Diminish the discoloration caused by scars, certain skin disorders, and age spots by applying lemon juice to the

discolored area. It may be helpful to apply the lemon juice at bedtime and leave it on the skin overnight.

Use lemon juice on acne and blackheads to reduce the frequency and severity. If you leave lemon juice on the acne and blackheads overnight, be sure to wash it off in the morning.

Try lemon juice as a natural exfoliant; the citric acid acts as a gentle "skin peel" that removes the top layer of dead skin cells. This results in a smooth complexion when used regularly. It also helps brighten or lighten the skin, moisturizes and tones, and fights wrinkles.

Apple-Cider Vinegar

Apple-cider vinegar is often recommended as a treatment for age spots and warts and as a hair conditioner, and it helps balance the pH of your тkin and hair.

For age spots, use a mixture of one part vinegar to two parts water as a toner. You can also apply undiluted apple-cider vinegar directly to the spots. Preferably, you should do this several times a day for at least a month. Some people have even better results mixing the vinegar with either fresh orange juice or onion juice and applying it several times a day.

You can treat warts with apple-cider by soaking a small cotton ball in the vinegar and using tape or a bandage to keep the soaked cotton ball in contact with the wart for as long as possible. You can either do it in the morning and keep it on all day or do it before bed and wear it overnight.

Be aware that the warts may turn black before falling off.

Continue with the treatment for a further week, even if the wart looks to be gone, to make sure it doesn't return.

Try doing a rinse of apple-cider vinegar after you тhampoo instead of using conditioner. It makes your hair lustrous and soft without any harsh chemicals.

Strawberries

Did you know you can put strawberries directly on your face by muтshing them into a mask or rubbing them over your skin?

They combat oil, work as an antioxidant, and brighten your face.

They're also rich in vitamin C, which has amazing benefits for brightening and nourishing your skin. They also can be used to whiten your teeth!

Bananas

Bananas whose skins have a few brown spots are perfect for a face mask. This means your bananas are slightly soft and ripe.

Bananas exfoliate like crazy and give new life to a dull complexion. They also moisturize and are great for all types of skin. Mush it up (add a little honey if you'd like) and rub it on your face. Leave on for 10 minutes and rinse.

Almonds and Oats

Toss either almonds or whole oats into the food processor and turn them into a powder. Then you can add water and use them as a facial scrub. They moisturize, exfoliate, and cleanse.

Almonds are also rich in vitamin E, which has nourishing properties to soothe skin and promote wound-healing.

Instead of water, add some non-dairy milk and turn these scrubs into a luxurious way to soothe dry or sunburned skin. Rub gently on the skin, being careful not to be too abrasive.

Olive Oil

Olive oil is a centuries-old beauty staple. Moisturize your face with it, condition your hair with it, or add some salt to make the easiest hand scrub ever.

A good rule of thumb when buying olive oils (or any oilт, really): Go for extra virgin, expeller pressed, and organic when you can. They're higher in antioxidants, contain fewer chemicals, and aren't as "messed with" as more-processed kinds.

Aloe Vera

Aloe vera is one of the most nourishing plants on the planet for the skin.

It's an excellent moisturizer for the skin and helps to rejuvenate, hydrate, and keep your skin looking fresh.

Aloe vera has antimicrobial properties, making it ideal to treat acne.

It's an amazing natural antioxidant.

It's helpful in retaining skin's firmness, making it a great anti-aging skin cream.

Aloe vera gel or meat, from the whole leaf, is also known to reduce pain and inflammation both internally and externally. It's most helpful with sunburns, insect bites, rashes, eczema, and cuts and wounds.

Just pull off a leaf and cut it open, extract the gel, and moisturize away!

Chapter 9:   Breakfasts

1. Tasty Oatmeal Muffins

Preparation time: 10 minutes

Cooking time: 20 minutes

Servings: 12

Ingredients:

½ cup of hot water

½ cup of raisins

¼ cup of ground flaxseed

2 cups of rolled oats

¼ teaspoon of sea salt

½ cup of walnuts

¼ teaspoon of baking soda

1 banana

2 tablespoons of cinnamon

¼ cup of maple syrup

Directions:

Whisk the flaxseed with water and allow the mixture to sit for about 5 minutes.

In a food processor, blend all the ingredients along with the flaxseed mix. Blend everything for 30 seconds, but do not create a smooth substance. To create rough-textured cookies, you need to have a semi-coarse batter.

Put the batter in cupcake liners and place them in a muffin tin. As this is an oil-free recipe, you will need cupcake liners. Bake everything for about 20 minutes at 350 degrees.

Enjoy the freshly-made cookies with a glass of warm milk.

Nutrition: Calories: 133, Fats 2 g, Carbohydrates 27 g, Protein 3 g

2. Omelette with Chickpea Flour

Preparation time: 10 minutes

Cooking time: 20 minutes

Serving: 1

Ingredients:

½ teaspoon, onion powder

¼ teaspoon, black pepper

1 cup, chickpea flour

½ teaspoon, garlic powder

½ teaspoon, baking soda

¼ teaspoon, white pepper

1/3 cup, nutritional yeast

3 finely chopped green onions

4 ounces, sautéed mushrooms

Directions:

In a small bowl, mix the onion powder, white pepper, chickpea flour, garlic powder, black and white pepper, baking soda, and nutritional yeast.

Add 1 cup of water and create a smooth batter.

On medium heat, put a frying pan and add the batter just like the way you would cook pancakes.

On the batter, sprinkle some green onion and mushrooms. Flip the omelet and cook evenly on both sides.

Once both sides are cooked, serve the omelet with spinach, tomatoes, hot sauce, and salsa.

Nutrition: Calories: 150, Fats 1.9 g, Carbohydrates 24.4 g, Proteins 10.2 g

3. White Sandwich Bread

Preparation time: 10 minutes

Cooking time: 20 minutes

Servings: 16

Ingredients:

1 cup warm water

2 tablespoons active dry yeast

4 tablespoons oil

2 ½ teaspoons salt

2 tablespoons raw sugar or 4 tablespoons maple syrup /agave nectar

1 cup warm almond milk or any other nondairy milk of your choice

6 cups all-purpose flour

Directions:

Add warm water, yeast and sugar into a bowl and stir. Set aside for 5 minutes or until lots of tiny bubbles are formed, sort of frothy.

Add flour and salt into a mixing bowl and stir. Pour the oil, yeast mix and milk and mix into dough. If the dough is too hard, add a little water, a tablespoon at a time and mix well each time. If the dough is too sticky, add more flour, a tablespoon at a time. Knead the dough for 8 minutes until soft and supple. You can use your hands or use the dough hook attachment of the stand mixer.

Now spray some water on top of the dough. Keep the bowl covered with a towel. Let it rest until it doubles in size.

Remove the dough from the bowl and place on your countertop. Punch the dough.

Line a loaf pan with parchment paper. You can also grease with ome oil if you prefer. You can use 2 smaller loaf pans if you want to make smaller loaves, like I did.

Place the dough in the loaf pan. Now spray some more water on top of the dough. Keep the loaf pan covered with a towel. Let it rest until the dough doubles in size.

Bake in a preheated oven at 370° F for about 40 – 50 minutes or a toothpick when inserted in the center of the bread comes out without any particles stuck on it.

Let it cool to room temperature.

Cut into 16 equal slices and use as required. Store in a breadbox at room temperature.

Nutrition: Calories 209, Fat 4 g, Carbohydrate 35 g, Protein 1 g

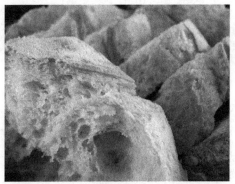

4. A Toast to Remember

Preparation time: 10 minutes

Cooking time: 15 minutes

Servings: 4

Ingredients:

1 can, black beans

Pinch, sea salt

2 pieces, whole-wheat toast

¼ teaspoon, chipotle spice

Pinch, black pepper

1 teaspoon, garlic powder

1 freshly juiced lime

1 freshly diced avocado

¼ cup, corn

3 tablespoons, finely diced onion

½ freshly diced tomato

Fresh cilantro

Directions:

Mix the chipotle spice with the beans, salt, garlic powder, and pepper. Stir in the lime juice.

Boil all of these until you have a thick and starchy mix.

In a bowl, mix the corn, tomato, avocado, red onion, cilantro, and juice from the rest of the lime. Add some pepper and salt.

Toast the bread and first spread the black bean mixture followed by the avocado mix.

Take a bite of wholesome goodness!

Nutrition: Calories: 290, Fats 9 g, Carbohydrates 44 g, Proteins 12 g

5. Tasty Panini

Preparation time: 5 minutes

Cooking time: 0 minutes

Serving: 1

Ingredients:

¼ cup, hot water

1 tablespoon, cinnamon

¼ cup, raisins

2 teaspoons, cacao powder

1 ripe banana

2 slices, whole-grain bread

¼ cup, natural peanut butter

Directions:

In a bowl, mix the cinnamon, hot water, raisins, and cacao powder.

Spread the peanut butter on the bread.

Cut the bananas and put them on the toast.

Mix the raisin mixture in a blender and spread it on the sandwich.

Nutrition: Calories: 850, Fats 34 g, Carbohydrates 112 g, Proteins 27 g

6. Tasty Oatmeal and Carrot Cake

Preparation time: 10 minutes

Cooking time: 10 minutes

Serving: 1

Ingredients:

1 cup, water

½ teaspoon, cinnamon

1 cup, rolled oats

Salt

¼ cup, raisins

½ cup, shredded carrots

1 cup, non-dairy milk

¼ teaspoon, allspice

½ teaspoon, vanilla extract

Toppings:

¼ cup, chopped walnuts

2 tablespoons, maple syrup

2 tablespoons, shredded coconut

Directions:

Put a small pot on low heat and bring the non-dairy milk, oats, and water to a simmer.

Now, add the carrots, vanilla extract, raisins, salt, cinnamon and allspice. You need to simmer all of the ingredients, but do not forget to stir them. You will know that they are ready when the liquid is fully absorbed into all of the ingredients (in about 7-10 minutes).

Transfer the thickened dish to bowls. You can drizzle some maple syrup on top or top them with coconut or walnuts.

Nutrition: Calories: 210, Fats 11.48 g, Carbohydrates 10.37 g, Proteins 3.8 g

7. Onion & Mushroom Tart with a Nice Brown Rice Crust

Preparation time 10 minutes

Cooking time 55 minutes

Serving: 1

Ingredients:

1 ½ pounds, mushrooms, button, portabella,

1 cup, short-grain brown rice

2 ¼ cups, water

½ teaspoon, ground black pepper

2 teaspoons, herbal spice blend

1 sweet large onion

7 ounces, extra-firm tofu

1 cup, plain non-dairy milk

2 teaspoons, onion powder

2 teaspoons, low-sodium soy

1 teaspoon, molasses

¼ teaspoon, ground turmeric

¼ cup, white wine

¼ cup, tapioca

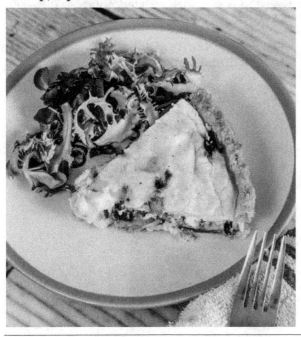

Directions:

Cook the brown rice and put it aside for later use.

Slice the onions into thin strips and sauté them in water until they are soft. Then, add the molasses, and cook them for a few minutes.

Next, sauté the mushrooms in water with the herbal spice blend. Once the mushrooms are cooked and they are soft, add the white wine or sherry. Cook everything for a few more minutes.

In a blender, combine milk, tofu, arrowroot, turmeric, and onion powder till you have a smooth mixture

On a pie plate, create a layer of rice, spreading evenly to form a crust. The rice should be warm and not cold. It will be easy to work with warm rice. You can also use a pastry roller to get an even crust. With your fingers, gently press the sides.

Take half of the tofu mixture and the mushrooms and spoon them over the tart dish. Smooth the level with your spoon.

Now, top the layer with onions followed by the tofu mixture. You can smooth the surface again with your spoon.

Sprinkle some black pepper on top.

Bake the pie at 3500 F for about 45 minutes. Toward the end, you can cover it loosely with tin foil. This will help the crust to remain moist.

Allow the pie crust to cool down, so that you can slice it. If you are in love with vegetarian dishes, there is no way that you will not love this pie.

Nutrition: Calories: 245.3, Fats 16.4 g, Proteins 6.8 g, Carbohydrates 18.3 g

8. Perfect Breakfast Shake

Preparation time: 5 minutes

Cooking time: 0 minutes

Servings: 2

Ingredients:

3 tablespoons, raw cacao powder

1 cup, almond milk

2 frozen bananas

3 tablespoons, natural peanut butter

Directions:

Use a powerful blender to combine all the ingredients.

Process everything until you have a smooth shake.

Enjoy a hearty shake to kickstart your day.

Nutrition: Calories: 330, Fats 15 g, Carbohydrates 41 g, Proteins 11 g

9. Beet Gazpacho

Preparation time: 10 minutes

Cooking time: 2 minutes

Servings: 4

Ingredients:

½ large bunch young beets with stems, roots and leaves

2 small cloves garlic, peeled,

Salt to taste

Pepper to taste

½ teaspoon liquid stevia

1 glass coconut milk kefir

1 teaspoon chopped dill

½ tablespoon canola oil

1 small red onion, chopped

1 tablespoon apple cider vinegar

2 cups vegetable broth or water

1 tablespoon chopped chives

1 scallion, sliced

Roasted baby potatoes

Directions:

Cut the roots and stems of the beets into small pieces. Thinly slice the beet greens.

Place a saucepan over medium heat. Add oil. When the oil is heated, add onion and garlic and cook until onion turns translucent.

Stir in the beets, roots and stem and cook for a minute.

Add broth, salt and water and cover with a lid. Simmer until tender.

Add stevia and vinegar and mix well. Taste and adjust the stevia and vinegar if required.

Turn off the heat. Blend with an immersion blender until smooth.

Place the saucepan back over it. When it begins to boil, add beet greens and cook for a minute. Turn off the heat.

Cool completely. Chill if desired.

Add rest of the ingredients and stir.

Serve in bowls with roasted potatoes if desired.

Nutrition: Calories 101, Fats 5 g, Carbohydrates 14 g, Proteins 2 g

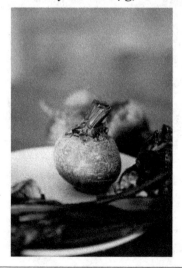

10.   Vegetable Rice

Preparation time: 7 minutes

Cooking time: 15 minutes

Servings: 4

Ingredients:

½ cup brown rice, rinsed

1 cup water

½ teaspoon dried basil

1 small onion, chopped

2 tablespoons raisins

5 ounces frozen peas, thawed

½ cup pecan halves, toasted

1 medium carrot, cut into matchsticks

4 green onions, cut into 1-inch pieces

1 tablespoon olive oil

½ teaspoon salt or to taste

½ teaspoon crushed red chili flakes or to taste

Ground pepper or to taste

Directions:

Place a small saucepan with water over medium heat.

When it begins to boil, add rice and basil. Stir.

When it again begins to boil, lower the heat and cover with a lid. Cook for 15 minutes until all the water is absorbed and rice is cooked. Add more water if you think the rice is not cooked well.

Meanwhile, place a skillet over medium high heat. Add carrots, raisins and onions and sauté until the vegetables are crisp as well as tender.

Stir in the peas, salt, pepper and chili flakes.

Add pecans and rice and stir.

Serve.

Nutrition: Calories 305, Fats 13 g, Carbohydrates 41 g, Proteins 8 g

11. Courgette Risotto

Preparation time: 10 minutes

Cooking time: 5 minutes

olive oil

finely chopped

rio rice

pped

pped rosemary

nely diced

fresh or frozen

etable stock

und pepper

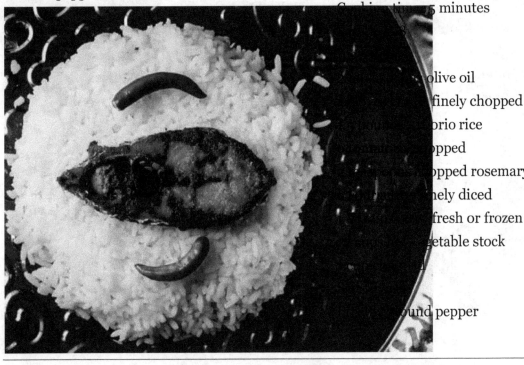

Directions:

Place a large heavy bottomed pan over medium heat. Add oil. When the oil is heated, add onion and sauté until translucent.

Stir in the tomatoes and cook until soft.

Next stir in the rice and rosemary. Mix well.

Add half the stock and cook until dry. Stir frequently.

Add remaining stock and cook for 3-4 minutes.

Add courgette and peas and cook until rice is tender. Add salt and pepper to taste.

Stir in the basil. Let it sit for 5 minutes.

Nutrition: Calories 406, Fats 5 g, Carbohydrates 82 g, Proteins 14 g

12. Country Breakfast Cereal

Preparation Time: 5 minutes

Cooking time: 40 minutes

Servings: 6

 Ingredients:

1 cup brown rice, uncooked

½ cup raisins, seedless

1 tsp cinnamon, ground

¼ Tbsp peanut butter

2 ¼ cups water

Honey, to taste

Nuts, toasted

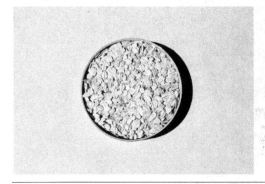

Directions:

Combine rice, butter, raisins, and cinnamon in a saucepan. Add 2 ¼ cups water. Bring to boil.

Simmer covered for 40 minutes until rice is tender.

Fluff with fork. Add honey and nuts to taste.

Nutrition: Calories 160 Carbohydrates 34 g Fats 1.5 g Protein 3 g

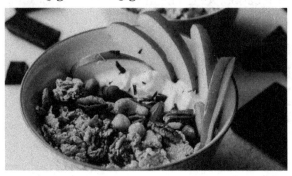

13. Oatmeal Fruit Shake

Preparation Time: 10 minutes

Cooking time: 0 minutes

Servings: 2

 Ingredients:

1 cup oatmeal, already prepared, cooled

1 apple, cored, roughly chopped

1 banana, halved

1 cup baby spinach

2 cups coconut water

2 cups ice, cubed

½ tsp ground cinnamon

1 tsp pure vanilla extract

Directions:

Add all ingredients to a blender.

Blend from low to high for several minutes until smooth.

Nutrition: Calories 270 Carbohydrates 58 g Fats 1.5 g Protein 5 g

14. Amaranth Banana Breakfast Porridge

Preparation Time: 10 minutes

Cooking time: 25 minutes

Servings: 8

Ingredients:

2 cup amaranth

2 cinnamon sticks

4 bananas, diced

2 Tbsp chopped pecans

4 cups water

Directions:

Combine the amaranth, water, and cinnamon sticks, and banana in a pot. Cover and let simmer around 25 minutes.

Remove from heat and discard the cinnamon. Places into bowls, and top with pecans.

Nutrition: Calories 330 Carbohydrates 62 g Fats 6 g Protein 10 g

15. Green Ginger Smoothie

Preparation time: 5 minutes

Cooking time: 5 minutes

Servings: 2

Ingredients:

1 banana

½ apple sliced

1 orange sliced and peeled

1 lemon juice

2 big spinach

1 tbsp. fresh ginger

½ cup almond milk

For the dressing: chia seeds, apple, raspberries

Directions:

Take a blender. Peel off and slice all fruits. Add banana, apple, orange, lime juice, ginger and spinach and blend them well until they turn smooth. Now add almond milk and pulse again for a few seconds. Pour the smoothie into glasses and serve. You can add chia seeds, apple or raspberries for a smoothie bowl. Store it up to 8-10 hours in the refrigerator.

Nutrition: Calories 330 Carbohydrates 62 g Fats 6 g Protein 10 g

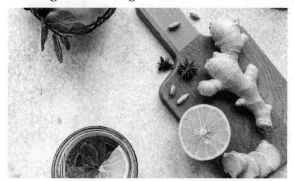

16. Orange Dream Creamsicle

Preparation time: 5 minutes

Cooking time: 5 minutes

Servings: 2

Ingredients:

1 orange, peeled

¼ cup vegan yogurt

2 tbsp. orange juice

¼ tsp vanilla extract

4 ice cubes

Directions:

In a blender, add orange, orange juice, vegan yogurt, vanilla extract and ice cubes. Blend all the ingredients well until smooth and well combined. Pour it into smoothie glasses and serve.

Nutrition: Calories 120 Carbohydrates 62 g Fats 6 g Protein 10g

17. Strawberry Limeade

Preparation time: 5 minutes

Cooking time: 5 minutes

Servings: 6

Ingredients:

2 cup strawberries

1 cup sugar or as per taste

7 cups of water

2 cup lemon juice

Sliced berries for garnish

Directions:

Take a small bowl, add sugar and water and put in microwave until dissolved. Now take a blender and add strawberries and a cup of water and blend well. Combine the strawberries puree with the sugar dissolve water and mix. Pour lime juice and water if required. Stir well and chill before serving. You can add berries on the top as garnishing.

Nutrition: Calories: 144, carbohydrates: 37g, sugar: 35g

18. Peanut Butter and Jelly Smoothie

Preparation time: 5 minutes

Cooking time: 5 minutes

Servings: 2

Ingredients:

1 cup frozen raspberries

1 cup frozen strawberries

1 serving collagen peptides

1 tbsp. peanut butter

¾ cup almond milk

Directions:

Take a blender. Add in raspberries, strawberries, peanut butter, collagen peptide and almond milk. Blend all ingredients until well combined. Add almond milk as per the required consistency. Pour into smoothie serving glasses and top up with the peanut butter or anything of your choice for dressing.

Nutrition: Calories: 251, fat: 11.1g, carbohydrates: 27.5g, proteins: 15.7g

19. Banana Almond Granola

Preparation time: 10 minutes

Cooking time: 20 Minutes

Servings: 21

Ingredients:

Organic rolled whole oats – 3 Cups

Raw Almond – ½ Cup, chopped

Sunflower seeds – ½ Cup, raw

Vanilla Extract – ½ teaspoon

Sea salt – 1/8 teaspoon

Coconut oil – 3 tablespoons, organic

Honey – 3 tablespoons, Raw

Banana – 2, ripe, small pieces

Directions:

Preheat the oven at 400F. Take a baking tray and line it with baking sheet. In a bowl, combine almonds, salt, vanilla and oats. In another small ball, combine honey, coconut oil (at room temperature), and bananas. Mash the bananas to make a smooth mixture. Now, add this banana mixture to the former dry mixture, combine until all ingredients coat each other well. Spread this mixture, granola, on the baking tray evenly. Place the tray into the preheated oven and bake it for at least 20 minutes. Check at 10 minutes interval, turn the granola upside down with the help of a spoon. Cool it down and store in a container for later use

Nutrition: Calories: 110 kcal; Fat: 5.4g; Carbohydrates: 14.2g; Sodium: 10.6mg; Protein: 2.9g

Chapter 10: Soups, Salads, and Sides

20. Spinach Soup with Dill and Basil

Preparation time: 10 minutes

Cooking time: 25 minutes

Servings: 8

Ingredients:

1 pound peeled and diced potatoes

1 tablespoon minced garlic

1 teaspoon dry mustard

6 cups vegetable broth

20 ounces chopped frozen spinach

2 cups chopped onion

1 ½ tablespoons salt

½ cup minced dill

1 cup basil

½ teaspoon ground black pepper

Directions:

Whisk onion, garlic, potatoes, broth, mustard, and salt in a pand cook it over medium flame. When it starts boiling, low down the heat and cover it with the lid and cook for 20 minutes. Add the remaining ingredients in it and blend it and cook it for few more minutes and serve it.

Nutrition: Carbohydrates 12g, protein 13g, fats 1g, calories 165.

21. Coconut Watercress Soup

Preparation time: 10 minutes

Cooking time: 20 minutes

Servings: 4

Ingredients:

1 teaspoon coconut oil

1 onion, diced

¾ cup coconut milk

Directions:

Preparing the ingredients.

Melt the coconut oil in a large pot over medium-high heat. Add the onion and cook until soft, about 5 minutes, then add the peas and the water. Bring to a boil, then lower the heat and add the watercress, mint, salt, and pepper.

Cover and simmer for 5 minutes. Stir in the coconut milk, and purée the soup until smooth in a blender or with an immersion blender.

Try this soup with any other fresh, leafy green—anything from spinach to collard greens to arugula to swiss chard.

Nutrition: calories: 178; protein: 6g; total fat: 10g; carbohydrates: 18g; fiber: 5g

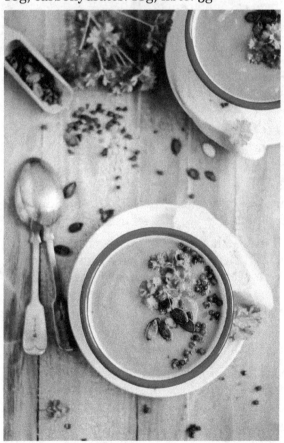

22.　Roasted Red Pepper and Butternut Squash Soup

Preparation time: 10 minutes

Cooking time: 45 minutes

Servings: 6

Ingredients:

1 small butternut squash

1 tablespoon olive oil

1 teaspoon sea salt

2 red bell peppers

1 yellow onion

1 head garlic

2 cups water, or vegetable broth

Zest and juice of 1 lime

1 to 2 tablespoons tahini

Pinch cayenne pepper

½ teaspoon ground coriander

½ teaspoon ground cumin

Toasted squash seeds (optional)

Directions:

Preparing the ingredients.

Preheat the oven to 350°f.

Prepare the squash for roasting by cutting it in half lengthwise, scooping out the seeds, and poking some holes in the flesh with a fork. Reserve the seeds if desired.

Rub a small amount of oil over the flesh and skin, then rub with a bit of sea salt and put the halves skin-side down in a large baking dish. Put it in the oven while you prepare the rest of the vegetables.

Prepare the peppers the exact same way, except they do not need to be poked.

Slice the onion in half and rub oil on the exposed faces. Slice the top off the head of garlic and rub oil on the exposed flesh.

After the squash has cooked for 20 minutes, add the peppers, onion, and garlic, and roast for another 20 minutes. Optionally, you can toast the squash seeds by putting them in the oven in a separate baking dish 10 to 15 minutes before the vegetables are finished.

Keep a close eye on them. When the vegetables are cooked, take them out and let them cool before handling them. The squash will be very soft when poked with a fork.

Scoop the flesh out of the squash skin into a large pot (if you have an immersion blender) or into a blender.

Chop the pepper roughly, remove the onion skin and chop the onion roughly, and squeeze the garlic cloves out of the head, all into the pot or blender. Add the water, the lime zest and juice, and the tahini. Purée the soup, adding more water if you like, to your desired consistency. Season with the salt, cayenne, coriander, and cumin. Serve garnished with toasted squash seeds (if using).

Nutrition: calories: 156; protein: 4g; total fat: 7g; saturated fat: 11g; carbohydrates: 22g; fiber: 5g

23.　Tomato Pumpkin Soup

Preparation time: 25 minutes

Cooking time: 15 minutes

Servings: 4

Ingredients:

2 cups pumpkin, diced

1/2 cup tomato, chopped

1/2 cup onion, chopped

1 1/2 tsp curry powder

1/2 tsp paprika

2 cups vegetable stock

1 tsp olive oil

1/2 tsp garlic, minced

Directions:

In a saucepan, add oil, garlic, and onion and sauté for 3 minutes over medium heat.

Add remaining ingredients into the saucepan and bring to boil.

Reduce heat and cover and simmer for 10 minutes.

Puree the soup using a blender until smooth.

Stir well and serve warm.

Nutrition: calories 70; fat 2.7 g; carbohydrates 13.8 g; sugar 6.3 g; protein 1.9 g; cholesterol 0 mg

24. Cauliflower Spinach Soup

Preparation time: 45 minutes

Cooking time: 25 minutes

Servings: 5

Ingredients:

1/2 cup unsweetened coconut milk

5 oz fresh spinach, chopped

5 watercress, chopped

8 cups vegetable stock

1 lb cauliflower, chopped

Salt

Directions:

Add stock and cauliflower in a large saucepan and bring to boil over medium heat for 15 minutes.

Add spinach and watercress and cook for another 10 minutes.

Remove from heat and puree the soup using a blender until smooth.

Add coconut milk and stir well. Season with salt.

Stir well and serve hot.

Nutrition: calories 153; fat 8.3 g; carbohydrates 8.7 g; sugar 4.3 g; protein 11.9 g; cholesterol 0 mg

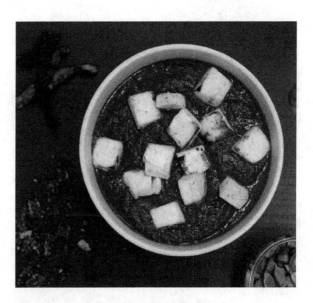

25. Avocado Mint Soup

Preparation time: 10 minutes

Cooking time: 10 minutes

Servings: 2

Ingredients:

1 medium avocado, peeled, pitted, and cut into pieces

1 cup coconut milk

2 romaine lettuce leaves

20 fresh mint leaves

1 tbsp fresh lime juice

1/8 tsp salt

Directions:

Add all ingredients into the blender and blend until smooth. Soup should be thick not as a puree.

Pour into the serving bowls and place in the refrigerator for 10 minutes.

Stir well and serve chilled.

Nutrition: calories 268; fat 25.6 g; carbohydrates 10.2 g; sugar 0.6 g; protein 2.7 g; cholesterol 0 mg

26. Creamy Squash Soup

Preparation time: 35 minutes

Cooking time: 22 minutes

Servings: 8

Ingredients:

3 cups butternut squash, chopped

1 ½ cups unsweetened coconut milk

1 tbsp coconut oil

1 tsp dried onion flakes

1 tbsp curry powder

4 cups water

1 garlic clove

1 tsp kosher salt

Directions:

Add squash, coconut oil, onion flakes, curry powder, water, garlic, and salt into a large saucepan. Bring to boil over high heat.

Turn heat to medium and simmer for 20 minutes.

Puree the soup using a blender until smooth. Return soup to the saucepan and stir in coconut milk and cook for 2 minutes.

Stir well and serve hot.

Nutrition: calories 146; fat 12.6 g; carbohydrates 9.4 g; sugar 2.8 g; protein 1.7 g; cholesterol 0 mg

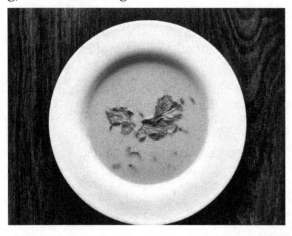

27. Cucumber Edamame Salad

Preparation time: 5 minutes

Cooking time: 8 minutes

Servings: 2

 Ingredients:

3 tbsp. Avocado oil

1 cup cucumber, sliced into thin rounds

½ cup fresh sugar snap peas, sliced or whole

½ cup fresh edamame

¼ cup radish, sliced

1 large avocado, peeled, pitted, sliced

1 nori sheet, crumbled

2 tsp. Roasted sesame seeds

1 tsp. Salt

Directions:

Bring a medium-sized pot filled halfway with water to a boil over medium-high heat.

Add the sugar snaps and cook them for about 2 minutes.

Take the pot off the heat, drain the excess water, transfer the sugar snaps to a medium-sized bowl and set aside for now.

Fill the pot with water again, add the teaspoon of salt and bring to a boil over medium-high heat.

Add the edamame to the pot and let them cook for about 6 minutes.

Take the pot off the heat, drain the excess water, transfer the soybeans to the bowl with sugar snaps and let them cool down for about 5 minutes.

Combine all ingredients, except the nori crumbs and roasted sesame seeds, in a medium-sized bowl.

Carefully stir, using a spoon, until all ingredients are evenly coated in oil.

Top the salad with the nori crumbs and roasted sesame seeds.

Transfer the bowl to the fridge and allow the salad to cool for at least 30 minutes.

Serve chilled and enjoy!

Nutrition: Calories 409 Carbohydrates 7.1 g Fats 38.25 g Protein 7.6 g

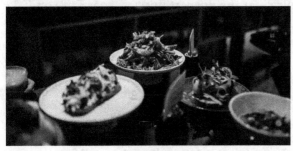

28. Best Broccoli Salad

Preparation time: 15 minutes

Chilling time: 1 hour

Servings: 8

Ingredients:

8 cups diced broccoli

¼ cup sunflower seeds

3 tablespoons apple cider vinegar

½ cup dried cranberries

1/3 cup cubed onion

1 cup mayonnaise

½ cup bacon bits

2 tablespoons sugar

½ teaspoon salt and ground black pepper

Directions:

In a bowl, mix vinegar, salt, pepper, mayonnaise, and sugar. Mix it well. In another bowl, mix all the remaining ingredients and pour the prepared mayonnaise dressing and mix it well. Before serving to refrigerate it for at least an hour.

Nutrition: Carbohydrates 17g, protein 6g, fats 26g, calories 317

29. Rainbow Orzo Salad

Preparation time: 10 minutes

Cooking time: 20 minutes

Servings: 1

Ingredients:

1 chopped onion

25g grated feta cheese

2 sliced bell peppers

1 tablespoon olive oil

6 sliced tomatoes

2 tablespoons chopped basil

25g orzo pasta

Directions:

Preheat the oven at 350f temperature. Prepare a baking sheet and place the onion and bell peppers and drizzle half olive oil. Bake it for around 15 minutes. Add tomatoes on it and bake for an additional 5 minutes. Meanwhile, cook the orzo according to the given directions on the pack and cool it. Now toss it with the baked vegetables and top it with cheese, basil and remaining oil and serve it.

Nutrition: Carbohydrates 52g, protein 13g, fats 18g, calories 422, sugar 30g.

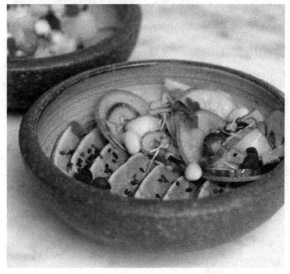

30. Broccoli Pasta Salad

Preparation time: 15 minutes

Chilling time: 30 minutes

Servings: 12

Ingredients:

1-pound cooked pasta

2 diced broccoli florets

1 chopped onion

1 cup grated cheese

12 ounce cooked and finely chopped bacon

¾ teaspoon salt

¾ teaspoon ground black pepper

1 cup mayonnaise

Directions:

Take a bowl and mix all the ingredients until all of them combined well. Cover it with the plastic wrap and place it in the refrigerator for at least 30 minutes and serve it. You can keep it in the refrigerator for 3 days.

Nutrition: Carbohydrates 36g, protein 14g, fats 29g, calories 461.

31. Eggplant & Roasted Tomato Farro Salad

Preparation time: 1 hour

Cooking time: 1 hour 30 minutes

Servings: 3

 Ingredients:

4 small eggplants

1 ½ cups chopped cherry tomatoes

¾ cup uncooked faro

1 tablespoon olive oil

1 minced garlic clove

½ cup rinsed and drained chickpeas

1 tablespoon basil

1 tablespoon arugula

½ teaspoon salt and ground black pepper

1 tablespoon vinegar

½ cup toasted pine nuts

Directions:

Preheat the oven at 300f temperature and prepare a baking sheet. Place cherry tomatoes on the baking liner and drizzle olive oil, salt, and black pepper on it and bake it for 30 to 35 minutes. Cook the faro in the salted water for 30 to 40 minutes. Slice the eggplant and salt it and leave it for 30 minutes. After that, rinse it with water and dry it kitchen towel. Now peeled and sliced the eggplants. Now place these slices on the baking liner and season it with salt, pepper and olive oil. Bake it for 15 to 20 minutes in the preheated oven at the 450f temperature. Flip the sides of eggplant and bake it for an additional 15 to 20 minutes. Bake the pine nuts for 5 minutes and sauté the garlic. Now mix all the ingredients in a bowl and serve it.

Nutrition: Carbohydrates 37g, protein 9g, fats 25g, calories 399.

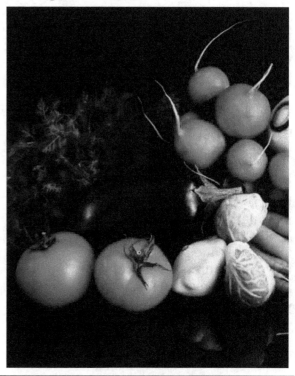

32. Garden Patch Sandwiches on Multigrain Bread

Preparation time: 15 minutes

Cooking time: 0 minutes

Servings: 4 sandwiches

Ingredients:

1pound extra-firm tofu, drained and patted dry

1 medium red bell pepper, finely chopped

1 celery rib, finely chopped

3 green onions, minced

1/4 cup shelled sunflower seeds

1/2 cup vegan mayonnaise, homemade or store-bought

1/2 teaspoon salt

1/2 teaspoon celery salt

1/4 teaspoon freshly ground black pepper

8 slices whole grain bread

4 (1/4-inch) slices ripe tomato

4 lettuce leaves

Directions:

Crumble the tofu and place it in a large bowl. Add the bell pepper, celery, green onions, and sunflower seeds. Stir in the mayonnaise, salt, celery salt, and pepper and mix until well combined.

Toast the bread, if desired. Spread the mixture evenly onto 4 slices of the bread. Top each with a tomato slice, lettuce leaf, and the remaining bread. Cut the sandwiches diagonally in half and serve.

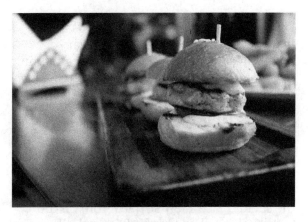

33. Garden Salad Wraps

Preparation time: 15 minutes

Cooking time: 10 minutes

Servings: 4 wraps

 Ingredients:

6 tablespoons olive oil

1-pound extra-firm tofu, drained, patted dry, and cut into 1/2-inch strips

1 tablespoon soy sauce

1/4 cup apple cider vinegar

1 teaspoon yellow or spicy brown mustard

1/2 teaspoon salt

1/4 teaspoon freshly ground black pepper

3 cups shredded romaine lettuce

3 ripe roma tomatoes, finely chopped

1 large carrot, shredded

1 medium english cucumber, peeled and chopped

1/3 cup minced red onion

1/4 cup sliced pitted green olives

4 (10-inch) whole-grain flour tortillas or lavash flatbread

Directions:

In a large skillet, heat 2 tablespoons of the oil over medium heat. Add the tofu and cook until golden brown, about 10 minutes.

Sprinkle with soy sauce and set aside to cool.

In a small bowl, combine the vinegar, mustard, salt, and pepper with the remaining 4 tablespoons oil, stirring to blend well. Set aside.

In a large bowl, combine the lettuce, tomatoes, carrot, cucumber, onion, and olives. Pour on the dressing and toss to coat.

To assemble wraps, place 1 tortilla on a work surface and spread with about one-quarter of the salad. Place a few strips of tofu on the tortilla and roll up tightly. Slice in half

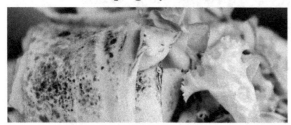

34. Marinated Mushroom Wraps

Preparation time: 15 minutes

Cooking time: 0 minutes

Servings: 2 wraps

Ingredients:

3 tablespoons soy sauce

3 tablespoons fresh lemon juice

1½ tablespoons toasted sesame oil

2 portobello mushroom caps, cut into ¼-inch strips

1 ripe hass avocado, pitted and peeled

2 cups fresh baby spinach leaves

1 medium red bell pepper, cut into ¼-inch strips

1 ripe tomato, chopped

Salt and freshly ground black pepper

Directions:

In a medium bowl, combine the soy sauce, 2 tablespoons of the lemon juice, and the oil.

Add the portobello strips, toss to combine, and marinate for 1 hour or overnight. Drain the mushrooms and set aside.

Mash the avocado with the remaining 1 tablespoon of lemon juice.

To assemble wraps, place 1 tortilla on a work surface and spread with some of the mashed avocado. Top with a layer of baby spinach leaves. In the lower third of each tortilla, arrange strips of the soaked mushrooms and some of the bell pepper strips. Sprinkle with the tomato and salt and black pepper to taste. Roll up tightly and cut in half diagonally. Repeat with the remaining ingredients and serve.

35. Tamari Toasted Almonds

Preparation time: 2 minutes

Cooking time: 8 minutes

Servings: ½ cup

Ingredients:

½ cup raw almonds, or sunflower seeds

2 tablespoons tamari, or soy sauce

1 teaspoon toasted sesame oil

Directions:

Preparing the ingredients.

Heat a dry skillet to medium-high heat, then add the almonds, stirring very frequently to keep them from burning. Once the almonds are toasted, 7 to 8 minutes for almonds, or 3 to 4 minutes for sunflower seeds, pour the tamari and sesame oil into the hot skillet and stir to coat.

You can turn off the heat, and as the almonds cool the tamari mixture will stick to and dry on the nuts.

Nutrition: calories: 89; total fat: 8g; carbs: 3g; fiber: 2g; protein: 4g

36. Nourishing Whole-Grain Porridge

Preparation time: 2 hours and 10 minutes

Cooking time: 2 hours

Servings: 4

Ingredients:

3/4 cup of steel-cut oats, rinsed and soaked overnight

3/4 cup of whole barley, rinsed and soaked overnight

1/2 cup of cornmeal

1 teaspoon of salt

3 tablespoons of brown sugar

1 cinnamon stick, about 3 inches long

1 teaspoon of vanilla extract, unsweetened

4 1/2 cups of water

Directions:

Using a 6-quarts slow cooker, place all the ingredients and stir properly.

Cover it with the lid, plug in the slow cooker and let it cook for 2 hours or until grains get soft, while stirring halfway through.

Serve the porridge with fruits.

Nutrition: Calories: 129 Cal, Carbohydrates:22g, Protein:5g, Fats:2g, Fiber:4g.

37. Pungent Mushroom Barley Risotto

Preparation time: 3 hours and 30 minutes

Cooking time: 3 hours and 9 minutes

Servings: 4

Ingredients:

1 1/2 cups of hulled barley, rinsed and soaked overnight

8 ounces of carrots, peeled and chopped

1 pound of mushrooms, sliced

1 large white onion, peeled and chopped

3/4 teaspoon of salt

1/2 teaspoon of ground black pepper

4 sprigs thyme

1/4 cup of chopped parsley

2/3 cup of grated vegan Parmesan cheese

1 tablespoon of apple cider vinegar

2 tablespoons of olive oil

1 1/2 cups of vegetable broth

Directions:

Place a large non-stick skillet pan over a medium-high heat, add the oil and let it heat until it gets hot.

Add the onion along with 1/4 teaspoon of each the salt and black pepper.

Cook it for 5 minutes or until it turns golden brown.

Then add the mushrooms and continue cooking for 2 minutes.

Add the barley, thyme and cook for another 2 minutes.

Transfer this mixture to a 6-quarts slow cooker and add the carrots, 1/4 teaspoon of salt, and the vegetable broth.

Stir properly and cover it with the lid.

Plug in the slow cooker, let it cook for 3 hours at the high heat setting or until the grains absorb all the cooking liquid and the vegetables get soft.

Remove the thyme sprigs, pour in the remaining ingredients except for parsley and stir properly.

Pour in the warm water and stir properly until the risotto reaches your desired state.

Add the seasoning, then garnish it with parsley and serve.

Nutrition: Calories:321 Cal, Carbohydrates:48g, Protein:12g, Fats:10g, Fiber:11g.

Chapter 11: Entrées

38.   Black Bean Dip

Preparation time: 1 hour and 30 minutes

Cooking time: 1 hour

Servings: 10

Ingredients:

2 15-ounce cans black beans, rinsed and drained

1 jalapeno pepper, seeded and minced

½ of a red bell pepper, seeded and diced

½ of a yellow bell pepper, seeded and diced

½ of s small red onion, diced

1 cup fresh cilantro, finely chopped

Zest of 1 lime

Juice of 1 lime

1 10-ounce can Ro*tel, drained

½ teaspoon Kosher salt

¼ teaspoon ground black pepper

Directions:

In a large bowl, combine the garlic, green onions, beans, jalapeno, red and yellow bell pepper, onion, cilantro and mix together well.

Add the lime zest and juice, Ro-tel, salt and pepper and mix. Adjust seasoning to your own taste.

Refrigerate for at one hour, minimum, before serving, so the flavors have time to blend. Serve with wheat tortilla slices that have been crisped in the oven or with wheat or sesame crackers.

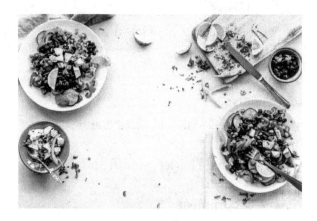

39.   Cannellini Bean Cashew Dip

Preparation time: 1 hour

Cooking time: 1 hour

Servings: 8

Ingredients:

1 15-ounce can cannellini beans, rinsed and drained

½ cup raw cashews

1 clove garlic, smashed

2 tablespoons diced, red bell pepper

½ teaspoon sea salt

¼ teaspoon cayenne pepper

4 teaspoons lemon juice

2 tablespoons water

Dill sprigs or weed for garnish

Directions:

Place the beans, cashews, garlic and bell pepper in the food processor and pulse several times to break it up.

Add the salt, cayenne, lemon juice and water and process until smooth.

Scrape into a bowl, cover and refrigerate for at least an hour before serving.

Garnish with fresh dill and serve with vegetables, crackers or pita chips.

40.   Cauliflower Popcorn

Preparation time: 1 day and 1 hour

Cooking time: 1 day

Servings: 2

Ingredients:

¼ cup sun-dried tomatoes

¾ cup dates

2 heads cauliflower

½ cup water

2 tablespoons raw tahini

1 tablespoon apple cider vinegar

2 teaspoons onion powder

2 teaspoons garlic powder

1 teaspoon ground cayenne pepper

2 tablespoons nutritional yeast (optional)

Directions:

Cover the sun-dried tomatoes warm water and let them soak for an hour.

If the dates are not soft and fresh, soak them in warm water for an hour in another bowl.

Cut the cauliflower in very small, bite-sized pieces then set aside.

Put the drained tomatoes and dates in a blender along with the water, tahini, apple cider vinegar, onion powder, garlic powder, cayenne pepper, nutritional yeast and turmeric. Blend into a thick, smooth consistency.

Pour this mixture into the bowl, atop the cauliflower and mix so that all the pieces are coated.

Place the cauliflower in the dehydrator and spread it out to make a single layer. Sprinkle with a little sea salt and set for 115 degrees, Fahrenheit for 12 to 24 hours or until it becomes exactly as crunchy as you like it. I let mine go for 15 to 16 hours, but the time will vary based on your taste preference as well as the ambient humidity.

Store in an airtight container until serving.

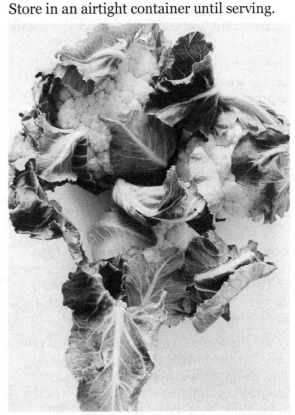

41.Cinnamon Apple Chips with Dip

Preparation time: 3 hours and 30 minutes

Cooking time: 3 hours

Servings: 2

Ingredients:

1 cup raw cashews

2 apples, thinly sliced

1 lemon

1½ cups water, divided

Cinnamon plus more to dust the chips

Another medium cored apple quartered

1 tablespoon honey or agave

1 teaspoon cinnamon

¼ teaspoon sea salt

Directions:

Place the cashews in a bowl of warm water, deep enough to cover them and let them soak overnight.

Preheat the oven to 200 degrees, Fahrenheit. Line two baking sheets with parchment paper.

Juice the lemon into a large glass bowl and add two cups of the water. Place the sliced apples in the water as you cut them and when done, swish them around and drain.

Spread the apple slices across the baking sheet in a single layer and sprinkle with a little cinnamon. Bake for 90 minutes.

Remove the slices from the oven and flip each of them over. Put them back in the oven and bake for another 90 minutes, or until they are crisp. Remember, they will get crisper as they cool.

While the apple slices are cooking, drain the cashews and put them in a blender, along with the quartered apple, the honey, a teaspoon of cinnamon and a half cup of the remaining water. Process until thick and creamy. I like to refrigerate my dip for about an hour to chill, before serve alongside the room temperature apple slices.

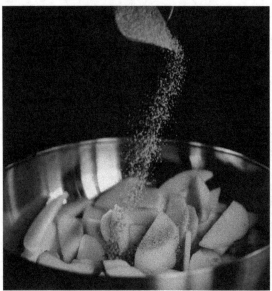

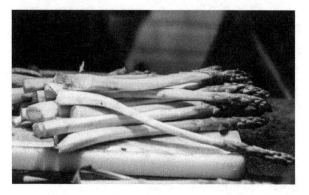

42.　Crunchy Asparagus Spears

Preparation time: 25 minutes

Cooking time: 25 minutes

Servings: 4

Ingredients:

1 bunch asparagus spears (about 12 spears)

¼ cup nutritional yeast

2 tablespoons hemp seeds

1 teaspoon garlic powder

¼ teaspoon paprika (or more if you like paprika)

⅛ teaspoon ground pepper

¼ cup whole-wheat breadcrumbs

Juice of ½ lemon

Directions:

Preheat the oven to 350 degrees, Fahrenheit. Line a baking sheet with parchment paper.

Wash the asparagus, snapping off the white part at the bottom. Save it for making vegetable stock.

Mix together the nutritional yeast, hemp seed, garlic powder, paprika, pepper and breadcrumbs.

Place asparagus spears on the baking sheets giving them a little room in between and sprinkle with the mixture in the bowl.

Bake for up to 25 minutes, until crispy.

Serve with lemon juice if desired.

43. Cucumber Bites with Chive and Sunflower Seeds

Preparation time: 5 minutes

Cooking time: 5 minutes

Servings: 2

Ingredients:

1 cup raw sunflower seed

½ teaspoon salt

½ cup chopped fresh chives

1 clove garlic, chopped

2 tablespoons red onion, minced

2 tablespoons lemon juice

½ cup water (might need more or less)

4 large cucumbers

Directions:

Place the sunflower seeds and salt in the food processor and process to a fine powder. It will take only about 10 seconds.

Add the chives, garlic, onion, lemon juice and water and process until creamy, scraping down the sides frequently. The mixture should be very creamy; if not, add a little more water.

Cut the cucumbers into 1½-inch coin-like pieces.

Spread a spoonful of the sunflower mixture on top and set on a platter. Sprinkle more chopped chives on top and refrigerate until ready to serve.

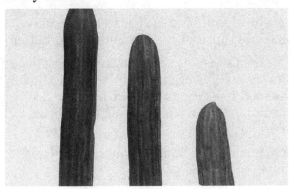

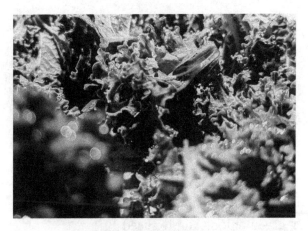

44. Garlicky Kale Chips

Preparation time: 1 hour and 30 min

Cooking time: 1 hour

Servings: 2

Ingredients:

4 cloves garlic

1 cup olive oil

8 to 10 cups fresh kale, chopped

1 tablespoon of garlic-flavored olive oil

½ teaspoon garlic salt

½ teaspoon pepper

1 pinch red pepper flakes (optional)

Directions:

Peel and crush the garlic clove and place it in a small jar with a lid. Pour the olive oil over the top, cover tightly and shake. This will keep in the refrigerator for several days. When you're ready to use it, strain out the garlic and retain the oil.

Preheat the oven to 175 degrees, Fahrenheit.

Spread out the kale on a baking sheet and drizzle with the olive oil. Sprinkle with garlic salt, pepper and red pepper flakes.

Bake for an hour, remove from the oven and let the chips cool.

Store in an airtight container if you don't plan to eat them right away.

45. Hummus-stuffed Baby Potatoes

Preparation time: 30 minutes

Cooking time: 30 minutes

Servings: 2

Ingredients:

12 small red potatoes, walnut-sized or slightly larger

Hummus

2 green onions, thinly sliced

¼ teaspoon paprika, for garnish

Directions:

Place two to three inches of water in a saucepan, set a steamer inside and bring the water to a boil.

Place the whole potatoes in the steamer basket and steam for about 20 minutes or until soft. Keep the pan from boiling dry by adding additional hot water as needed.

Dump the potatoes into a colander and run cold water over them until they can be handled.

Cut each potato open and scoop out most of the pulp, leaving the skin and a thin layer of potato intact.

Mix the hummus with most of the green onions (keep enough for garnish) and spoon a little into the area where the potato has been scooped out.

Sprinkle each filled potato half with paprika and serve.

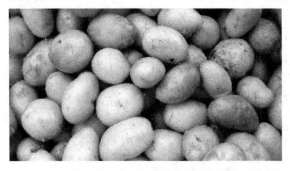

46. Homemade Trail Mix

Preparation time: 20 minutes

Cooking time: 20 minutes

Servings: 2

Ingredients:

½ cup uncooked old-fashioned oatmeal

½ cup chopped dates

2 cups whole grain cereal

¼ cup raisins

¼ cup almonds

¼ cup walnuts

Directions:

Mix all the ingredients in a large bowl.

Place in an airtight container until ready to use.

47. Nut Butter Maple Dip

Preparation time: 1 hour

Cooking time: 1 hour

Servings:

Ingredients:

½ tablespoon ground flaxseed

1 teaspoon ground cinnamon

½ tablespoon maple syrup

2 tablespoons cashew milk

¾ cups crunchy, unsweetened peanut butter

Directions:

In a bowl, combine the flaxseed, cinnamon, maple syrup, cashew milk and peanut butter.

Use a fork to mix everything in. I stir it like I'm scrambling eggs. The mixture should be creamy. If it's too runny, add a little more peanut butter; if it's too thick, add a little more cashew milk.

Refrigerate for about an hour, covered and serve.

48. Oven Baked Sesame Fries

Preparation time: 30 minutes

Cooking time: 30 minutes

Servings: 4

Ingredients:

1 pound Yukon Gold potatoes, skins on and cut into wedges

2 tablespoons sesame seeds

1 tablespoon potato starch

1 tablespoon sesame oil

Salt to taste

Black pepper to taste

Directions:

Preheat the oven to 425 degrees, Fahrenheit and cover a baking sheet or two with parchment paper.

Cut the potatoes and place in a large bowl.

Add the sesame seeds, potato starch, sesame oil, salt and pepper.

Toss with your hands and make sure all the wedges are coated. Add more sesame seeds or oil if needed.

Spread the potato wedges on the baking sheets with some room between each wedge.

Bake for 15 minutes, flip the wedges over and then return them to the oven for 10 to 15 more minutes, until they look golden and crispy.

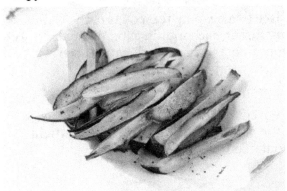

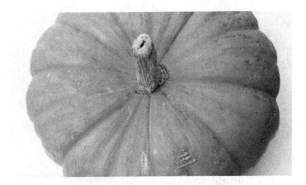

49. Pumpkin Orange Spice Hummus

Preparation time: 30 minutes

Cooking time: 30 minutes

Servings: 3

Ingredients:

1 cup canned, unsweetened pumpkin puree

1 16-ounce can garbanzo beans, rinsed and drained

1 tablespoon apple cider vinegar

1 tablespoon maple syrup

¼ cup tahini

1 tablespoon fresh orange juice

½ teaspoon orange zest and additional zest for garnish

⅛ teaspoon ground cinnamon

⅛ teaspoon ground ginger

⅛ teaspoon ground nutmeg

¼ teaspoon salt

Directions:

Pour the pumpkin puree and garbanzo beans into a food processor and pulse to break up.

Add the vinegar, syrup, tahini, orange juice and orange zest pulse a few times.

Add the cinnamon, ginger, nutmeg and salt and process until smooth and creamy.

Serve in a bowl sprinkled with more orange zest with wheat crackers alongside.

50. Quick English Muffin Mexican Pizzas

Preparation time: 30 minutes

Cooking time: 15 minutes

Servings:

Ingredients:

2 whole-wheat English muffins separated

⅓ cup tomato salsa

¼ cup refried beans

1 small jalapeno, seeded and sliced

¼ cup onion, sliced

2 tablespoons diced plum or cherry tomato

⅓ cup vegan cheese shreds (pepper jack is really tasty!)

Directions:

Preheat the oven to 400 degrees, Fahrenheit and cover a baking sheet with foil. The foil makes the crust crispier.

Separate the English muffin and spread on some salsa and refried beans.

Place some of the jalapenos and onions on top and sprinkle the cheese over all.

Place on the baking sheet and bake for 10 to 15 minutes or until brown. You can turn on the broiler for a minute or two to melt the cheese.

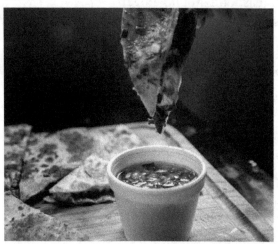

51. Quinoa Trail Mix Cups

Preparation time: 30 minutes

Cooking time: 30 minutes

Servings: 16

Ingredients:

2 tablespoons ground flaxseed

⅓ cup unsweetened soy milk

1 cup old-fashioned rolled oats

1 cup cooked and cooled quinoa

¼ cup brown sugar

1 teaspoon ground cinnamon

¼ teaspoon salt

¼ cup pumpkin or sunflower seeds

¼ cup shredded coconut

½ cup almonds

½ cup raisins or dried cherries/cranberries

Directions:

Whisk the flaxseed and milk together in a small bowl and set aside for 10 minutes so the seed can absorb the milk.

Preheat the oven to 350 degrees, Fahrenheit and coat a muffin tin with coconut oil.

In a large bowl, mix the oats, quinoa, brown sugar, cinnamon, salt, pumpkin seeds, coconut, almonds and raisins.

Stir in the flaxseed and milk mixture and combine thoroughly.

Place two heaping teaspoons of the trail mix mixture in each muffin cup. When done, wet your fingers and press down on each muffin cup to compact the trail mix.

Bake for 12 minutes.

Cool completely before removing and each little cup will fall out. Store in an airtight container.

Chapter 12: Smoothies and Beverages

52. Fruity Smoothie

Preparation Time: 10 Minutes

Cooking time: 0 minute

Servings: 1

Ingredients:

¾ cup soy yogurt

½ cup pineapple juice

1 cup pineapple chunks

1 cup raspberries, sliced

1 cup blueberries, sliced

Direction:

Process the ingredients in a blender.

Chill before serving.

Nutrition: Calories 279, Total Fat 2 g, Saturated Fat 0 g Cholesterol 4 mg, Sodium 149 mg, Total Carbohydrate 56 g Dietary Fiber 7 g, Protein 12 g, Total Sugars 46 g Potassium 719 mg

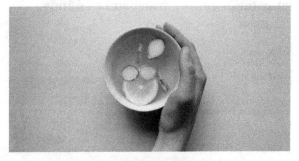

53. Energizing Ginger Detox Tonic

Preparation time: 15 minutes

Cooking time: 10 minutes

Servings: 2

Ingredients:

1/2 teaspoon of grated ginger, fresh

1 small lemon slice

1/8 teaspoon of cayenne pepper

1/8 teaspoon of ground turmeric

1/8 teaspoon of ground cinnamon

1 teaspoon of maple syrup

1 teaspoon of apple cider vinegar

2 cups of boiling water

Directions:

Pour the boiling water into a small saucepan, add and stir the ginger, then let it rest for 8 to 10 minutes, before covering the pan.

Pass the mixture through a strainer and into the liquid, add the cayenne pepper, turmeric, cinnamon and stir properly.

Add the maple syrup, vinegar, and lemon slice.

Add and stir an infused lemon and serve immediately.

Nutrition: Calories:80 Cal, Carbohydrates:0g, Protein:0g, Fats:0g, Fiber:0g.

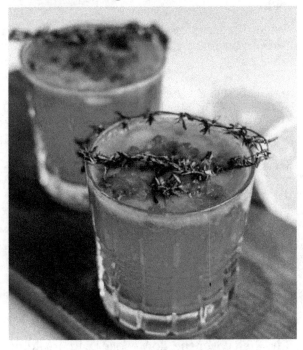

54.   Warm Spiced Lemon Drink

Preparation time: 2 hours and 10 minutes

Cooking time: 2 hours

Servings: 12

Ingredients:

1 cinnamon stick, about 3 inches long

1/2 teaspoon of whole cloves

2 cups of coconut sugar

4 fluid of ounce pineapple juice

1/2 cup and 2 tablespoons of lemon juice

12 fluid ounce of orange juice

2 1/2 quarts of water

Directions:

Pour water into a 6-quarts slow cooker and stir the sugar and lemon juice properly.

Wrap the cinnamon, the whole cloves in cheesecloth and tie its corners with string.

Immerse this cheesecloth bag in the liquid present in the slow cooker and cover it with the lid.

Then plug in the slow cooker and let it cook on high heat setting for 2 hours or until it is heated thoroughly.

When done, discard the cheesecloth bag and serve the drink hot or cold.

Nutrition: Calories:15 Cal, Carbohydrates:3.2g, Protein:0.1g, Fats:0g, Fiber:0g.

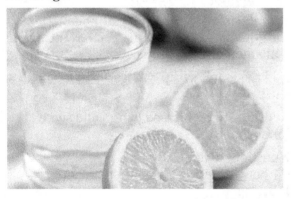

55.   Soothing Ginger Tea Drink

Preparation time: 2 hours and 15 minutes

Cooking time: 2 hours and 10 minutes

Servings: 8

Ingredients:

1 tablespoon of minced ginger root

2 tablespoons of honey

15 green tea bags

32 fluid ounce of white grape juice

2 quarts of boiling water

Directions:

Pour water into a 4-quarts slow cooker, immerse tea bags, cover the cooker and let stand for 10 minutes.

After 10 minutes, remove and discard tea bags and stir in remaining ingredients.

Return cover to slow cooker, then plug in and let cook at high heat setting for 2 hours or until heated through.

When done, strain the liquid and serve hot or cold.

Nutrition: Calories:45 Cal, Carbohydrates:12g, Protein:0g, Fats:0g, Fiber:0g.

56.   Nice Spiced Cherry Cider

Preparation time: 4 hours and 5 minutes

Cooking time: 4 hours

Servings: 16

Ingredients:

2 cinnamon sticks, each about 3 inches long

6-ounce of cherry gelatin

4 quarts of apple cider

Directions:

Using a 6-quarts slow cooker, pour the apple cider and add the cinnamon stick.

Stir, then cover the slow cooker with its lid.

Plug in the cooker and let it cook for 3 hours at the high heat setting or until it is heated thoroughly.

Then add and stir the gelatin properly, then continue cooking for another hour.

When done, remove the cinnamon sticks and serve the drink hot or cold.

Nutrition: , Calories:100 Cal, Carbohydrates:0g, Protein:0g, Fats:0g, Fiber:0g.

57. Fragrant Spiced Coffee

Preparation time: 3 hours and 10 minutes

Cooking time: 3 hours

Servings: 8

Ingredients:

4 cinnamon sticks, each about 3 inches long

1 1/2 teaspoons of whole cloves

1/3 cup of honey

2-ounce of chocolate syrup

1/2 teaspoon of anise extract

8 cups of brewed coffee

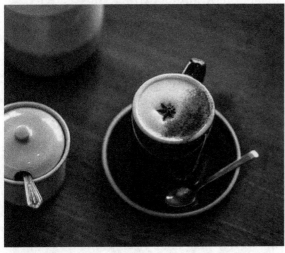

Directions:

Pour the coffee in a 4-quarts slow cooker and pour in the remaining ingredients except for cinnamon and stir properly.

Wrap the whole cloves in cheesecloth and tie its corners with strings.

Immerse this cheesecloth bag in the liquid present in the slow cooker and cover it with the lid.

Then plug in the slow cooker and let it cook on the low heat setting for 3 hours or until heated thoroughly.

When done, discard the cheesecloth bag and serve.

Nutrition: Calories:150 Cal, Carbohydrates:35g, Protein:3g, Fats:0g, Fiber:0g.

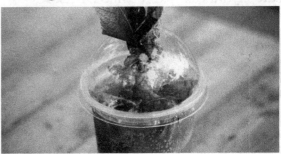

58. Tangy Spiced Cranberry Drink

Preparation time: 3 hours and 10 minutes

Cooking time: 3 hours

Servings: 14

Ingredients:

1 1/2 cups of coconut sugar

12 whole cloves

2 fluid ounce of lemon juice

6 fluid ounce of orange juice

32 fluid ounce of cranberry juice

8 cups of hot water

1/2 cup of Red Hot candies

Directions:

Pour the water into a 6-quarts slow cooker along with the cranberry juice, orange juice, and the lemon juice.

Stir the sugar properly.

Wrap the whole cloves in a cheese cloth, tie its corners with strings, and immerse it in the liquid present inside the slow cooker.

Add the red hot candies to the slow cooker and cover it with the lid.

Then plug in the slow cooker and let it cook on the low heat setting for 3 hours or until it is heated thoroughly.

When done, discard the cheesecloth bag and serve.

Nutrition: Calories:89 Cal, Carbohydrates:27g, Protein:0g, Fats:0g, Fiber:1g.

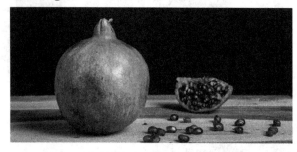

59.   Warm Pomegranate Punch

Preparation time: 3 hours and 15 minutes

Cooking time: 3 hours

Servings: 10

Ingredients:

3 cinnamon sticks, each about 3 inches long

12 whole cloves

1/2 cup of coconut sugar

1/3 cup of lemon juice

32 fluid ounce of pomegranate juice

32 fluid ounce of apple juice, unsweetened

16 fluid ounce of brewed tea

Directions:

Using a 4-quart slow cooker, pour the lemon juice, pomegranate, juice apple juice, tea, and then sugar.

Wrap the whole cloves and cinnamon stick in a cheese cloth, tie its corners with a string, and immerse it in the liquid present in the slow cooker.

Then cover it with the lid, plug in the slow cooker and let it cook at the low heat setting for 3 hours or until it is heated thoroughly.

When done, discard the cheesecloth bag and serve it hot or cold.

Nutrition: Calories:253 Cal, Carbohydrates:58g, Protein:7g, Fats:2g, Fiber:3g.

60.   Rich Truffle Hot Chocolate

Preparation time: 2 hours and 10 minutes

Cooking time: 2 hours

Servings: 4

Ingredients:

1/3 cup of cocoa powder, unsweetened

1/3 cup of coconut sugar

1/8 teaspoon of salt

1/8 teaspoon of ground cinnamon

1 teaspoon of vanilla extract, unsweetened

32 fluid ounce of coconut milk

Directions:

Using a 2 quarts slow cooker, add all the ingredients and stir properly.

Cover it with the lid, then plug in the slow cooker and cook it for 2 hours on the high heat setting or until it is heated thoroughly.

When done, serve right away.

Nutrition: Calories:67 Cal, Carbohydrates:13g, Protein:2g, Fats:2g, Fiber:2.3g.

61. Ultimate Mulled Wine

Preparation time: 35 minutes

Cooking time: 30 minutes

Servings: 6

Ingredients:

1 cup of cranberries, fresh

2 oranges, juiced

1 tablespoon of whole cloves

2 cinnamon sticks, each about 3 inches long

1 tablespoon of star anise

1/3 cup of honey

8 fluid ounce of apple cider

8 fluid ounce of cranberry juice

24 fluid ounce of red wine

Directions:

Using a 4 quarts slow cooker, add all the ingredients and stir properly.

Cover it with the lid, then plug in the slow cooker and cook it for 30 minutes on thee high heat setting or until it gets warm thoroughly.

When done, strain the wine and serve right away.

Nutrition: Calories:202 Cal, Carbohydrates:25g, Protein:0g, Fats:0g, Fiber:0g.

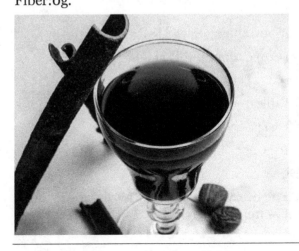

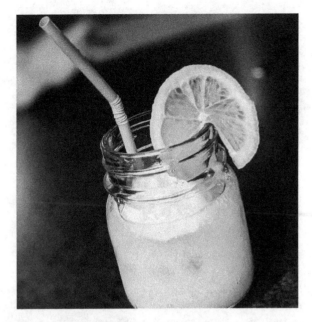

62.   Pleasant Lemonade

Preparation time: 3 hours and 15 minutes

Cooking time: 3 hours

Servings: 10 servings

Ingredients:

Cinnamon sticks for serving

2 cups of coconut sugar

1/4 cup of honey

3 cups of lemon juice. fresh

32 fluid ounce of water

Directions:

Using a 4-quarts slow cooker, place all the ingredients except for the cinnamon sticks and stir properly.

Cover it with the lid, then plug in the slow cooker and cook it for 3 hours on the low heat setting or until it is heated thoroughly.

When done, stir properly and serve with the cinnamon sticks.

Nutrition: Calories:146 Cal, Carbohydrates:34g, Protein:0g, Fats:0g, Fiber:0g.

63. Pineapple, Banana & Spinach Smoothie

Preparation Time: 10 Minutes

Cooking time: 0 minute

Servings: 1

Ingredients:

½ cup almond milk

¼ cup soy yogurt

1 cup spinach

1 cup banana

1 cup pineapple chunks

1 tbsp. chia seeds

Direction:

Add all the ingredients in a blender.

Blend until smooth.

Chill in the refrigerator before serving.

Nutrition: Calories 297, Total Fat 6 g, Saturated Fat 1 g, Cholesterol 4 mg   Sodium 145 mg, Total Carbohydrate 54 g, Dietary Fiber 10 g   Protein 13 g, Total Sugars 29g, Potassium 1038 mg

64. Kale & Avocado Smoothie

Preparation Time: 10 Minutes

Cooking time: 0 minute

Servings: 1

Ingredients:

1 ripe banana

1 cup kale

1 cup almond milk

¼ avocado

1 tbsp. chia seeds

2 tsp. honey

1 cup ice cubes

Direction:

Blend all the ingredients until smooth.

Nutrition: Calories 343 Total Fat 14 g Saturated Fat 2 g Cholesterol 0 mg   Sodium 199 mg   Total Carbohydrate 55 g   Dietary Fiber 12 g   Protein 6 g   Total Sugars 29 g Potassium 1051 mg

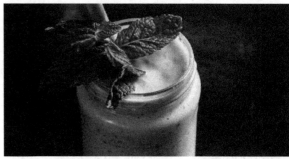

65. Coconut & Strawberry Smoothie

Preparation Time: 10 Minutes

Cooking Time: 0 minutes

Serves: 1

Calories: 278

Protein: 14 Grams

Fat: 2 Grams

Carbs: 57 Grams

Ingredients:

1 Cup Strawberries, Frozen & Thawed Slightly

1 Ripe Banana, Sliced & Frozen

½ Cup Coconut Milk, Light

½ Cup Vegan Yogurt

1 Tablespoon Chia Seeds

1 Teaspoon Lime juice, Fresh

4 Ice Cubes

Directions:

Blend everything together until smooth, and serve immediately.

66. Pumpkin Chia Smoothie

Preparation Time: 5 Minutes

Cooking Time: 0 minutes

Serves: 1

Calories: 726

Protein: 5.5 Grams

Fat: 69.8 Grams

Carbs: 15 Grams

Ingredients:

3 Tablespoons Pumpkin Puree

1 Tablespoon MCT Oil

¾ Cup Coconut Milk, Full Fat

½ Avocado, Fresh

1 Teaspoon Vanilla, Pure

½ Teaspoon Pumpkin Pie Spice

Directions:

Combine all ingredients together until blended.

67. Cantaloupe Smoothie Bowl

Preparation Time: 5 Minutes

Cooking Time: 0 minutes

Serves: 2

Calories: 135

Protein: 3 Grams

Fat: 1 Gram

Carbs: 32 Grams

Ingredients:

¾ Cup carrot Juice

4 Cps Cantaloupe, Frozen & Cubed

Mellon Balls or Berries to Serve

Pinch Sea Salt

Directions:

Blend everything together until smooth.

68. Berry & Cauliflower Smoothie

Preparation Time: 10 Minutes

Cooking Time: 0 minutes

Serves: 2

Calories: 149

Protein: 3 Grams

Fat: 3 Grams

Carbs: 29 Grams

Ingredients:

1 Cup Riced Cauliflower, Frozen

1 Cup Banana, Sliced & Frozen

½ Cup Mixed Berries, Frozen

2 Cups Almond Milk, Unsweetened

2 Teaspoons Maple syrup, Pure & Optional

Directions:

Blend until mixed well.

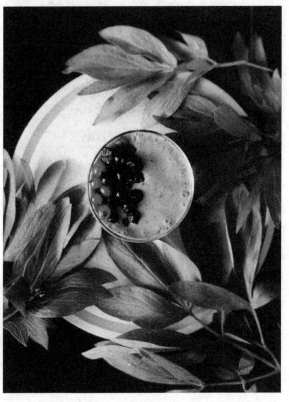

69.   Green Mango Smoothie

Preparation Time: 5 Minutes

Cooking Time: 0 minutes

Serves: 1

Calories: 417

Protein: 7.2 Grams

Fat: 2.8 Grams

Carbs: 102.8 Grams

Ingredients:

2 Cups Spinach

1-2 Cups Coconut Water

2 Mangos, Ripe, Peeled & Diced

Directions:

Blend everything together until smooth.

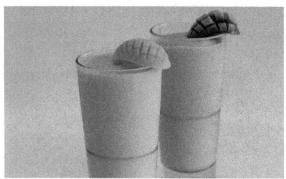

70.   Chia Seed Smoothie

Preparation Time: 5 Minutes

Cooking Time: 0 minutes

Serves: 3

Calories: 477

Protein: 8 Grams

Fat: 29 Grams

Carbs: 57 Grams

Ingredients:

¼ Teaspoon Cinnamon

1 Tablespoon Ginger, Fresh & Grated

Pinch Cardamom

1 Tablespoon Chia Seeds

2 Medjool Dates, Pitted

1 Cup Alfalfa Sprouts

1 Cup Water

1 Banana

½ Cup Coconut Milk, Unsweetened

Directions:

Blend everything together until smooth.

71. Mango Smoothie

Preparation Time: 5 Minutes

Cooking Time: 0 minutes

Serves: 3

Calories: 376

Protein: 5 Grams

Fat: 2 Grams

Carbs: 95 Grams

Ingredients:

1 Carrot, Peeled & Chopped

1 Cup Strawberries

1 Cup Water

1 Cup Peaches, Chopped

1 Banana, Frozen & sliced

1 Cup Mango, Chopped

Directions:

Blend everything together until smooth.

Snacks and Desserts

72.   Mango And Banana Shake

Preparation time: 10 mins

Cooking time: 0 mins

Servings: 2

Ingredients:

1 Banana, Sliced And Frozen

1 Cup Frozen Mango Chunks

1 Cup Almond Milk

1 Tbsp. Maple Syrup

1 Tsp Lime Juice

2-4 Raspberries For Topping

Mango Slice For Topping

Directions

In blender, pulse banana, mango with milk, maple syrup, lime juice until smooth but still thick

Add more liquid if needed.

Pour shake into 2 bowls.

Top with berries and mango slice.

Enjoy!

Nutrition: Protein: 5% 8 kcal Fat: 11% 18 kcal Carbohydrates: 85% 140 kcal

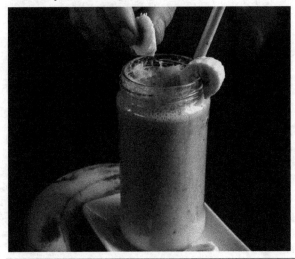

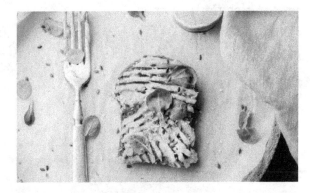

73.   Avocado Toast With Flaxseeds

Preparation time: 5 mins.

Cooking time: 0 mins

Servings: 3

Ingredients:

3 slice of whole grain bread

1 large avocado, ripe

¼ cup chopped parsley

1 tbsp. flax seeds

1 tbsp. sesame seeds

1 tbsp. lime juice

Directions:

First, toast your piece of bread.

Remove the avocado seed.

Slice half avocado and mash half avocado with fork in bowl.

Spread mashed avocado on 2 toasted bread.

Place avocado slice on 1 toast.

Top with flax seeds and sesame seeds.

Drizzle lime juice and chopped parsley on top.

Serve and enjoy!

Nutrition: Protein: 12% 31 kcal Fat: 49% 124 kcal Carbohydrates: 39% 98 kcal

74. Avocado Hummus

Preparation time: 10 mins

Cooking time:

Servings: 4

Ingredients

2 Ripe Avocados

½ Cup Coconut Cream

¼ Cup Sesame Paste

½ Lemon Juice

1 Tsp. Clove, Pressed

½ Tsp Ground Cumin

½ Tsp Salt

¼ Tsp Ground Black Pepper

Directions

Cut the avocado lengthways and remove seed from the fruit.

Put all ingredients in a blender or food processor and mix until thoroughly smooth.

Add more cream, lemon juice or water if you want to have a looser texture.

Adjust seasonings as needed.

Serve with naan and enjoy.

Nutrition: Protein: 6% 21 kcal Fat: 79% 289 kcal Carbohydrates: 16% 57 kcal

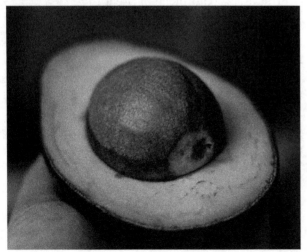

75. Plant Based Crispy Falafel

Preparation time: 20 mins

Cooking time: 30 mins

Servings: 8

Ingredients

1 tbsp. extra-virgin olive oil

1 cup dried chickpeas soaked for 24 hours in the refrigerator

1 cup cauliflower, chopped

½ cup red onion, chopped

½ cup packed fresh parsley

2 cloves garlic, quartered

1 tsp. sea salt

½ tsp. ground black pepper

½ tsp. ground cumin

¼ tsp. ground cinnamon

Directions

Preheat oven to 375° F.

In a food processor, mix chickpeas, cauliflower, onion, parsley, garlic, salt, pepper, cumin seeds, cinnamon, and olive oil until mixture is smooth.

Take 2 tbsps. of mixture and make the falafel into small patties.

Keep falafel on greased baking tray.

Bake falafel for about 25 to 30 minutes in preheated oven until golden brown from both sides.

Once cooked remove from oven.

Serve hot fresh vegetable salad and enjoy!

Nutrition: Protein: 16% 19 kcal Fat: 24% 29 kcal Carbohydrates: 60% 71 kcal

76. Waffles With Almond Flour

Preparation time: 15 mins

Cooking time: 15 mins

Servings: 4

Ingredients

1 cup almond milk

2 tbsps. chia seeds

2 tsp lemon juice

4 tbsps. coconut oil

1/2 cup almond flour

2 tbsps. maple syrup

Cooking spray or cooking oil

Directions

Mix coconut milk with lemon juice in a mixing bowl.

Leave it for 5-8 minutes on room temperature to turn it into butter milk.

Once coconut milk is turned into butter milk, add chai seeds into milk and whisk together.

Add other ingredients in milk mixture and mix well.

Preheat a waffle iron and spray it with coconut oil spray.

Pour 2 tbsp. of waffle mixture into the waffle machine and cook until golden.

Top with some berries and serve hot.

Enjoy with black coffee!

Nutrition: Protein: 5% 15 kcal Fat: 71% 199 kcal Carbohydrates: 23% 66 kcal

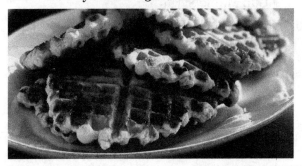

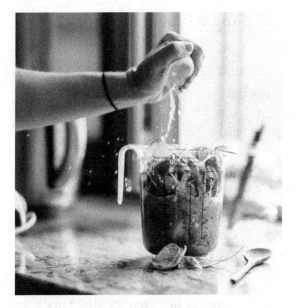

77. Mint & Avocado Smoothie

Preparation time: 10 mins

Cooking time: 0 minutes

Servings: 2

Ingredients

1 cup coconut water

1/2 lemon juice

½ cup cucumber

1 cup mint. fresh

1/2 medium size avocado

I/2 tsp maple syrup

1 cup ice

Directions

Place all ingredients into a blender, cover lid and blend until smooth.

Blend on high speed until smoothie has fluffy texture.

Pour smoothie in glass and top with mint leaves.

Serve and enjoy!

Nutrition: Protein: 6% 7 kcal Fat: 51% 64 kcal Carbohydrates: 44% 55 kcal

78. Simple Banana Fritters

Preparation time: 15 mins

Cooking time: 20 mins

Servings: 8

Ingredients

4 Bananas

3 Tbsps. Maple Syrup

¼ Tsp. Cinnamon Powder

¼ Tsp. Nutmeg

1 Cup Coconut Flour

Directions

Preheat oven to 350° F.

Mash the bananas in a large mixing bowl along with maple syrup, cinnamon, nutmeg powder and coconut flour.

Mix all the ingredients well.

Take 2 tbsps. mixture and make small 1-inch-thick fritters from this mixture.

Place fritters in greased baking tray.

Bake fritters in preheated oven for about 10-15 minutes until golden from both sides.

Once done, take them out of the oven.

Serve with coconut cream.

Enjoy!

Nutrition: Protein: 3% 3 kcal Fat: 28% 30 kcal Carbohydrates: 69% 75 kcal

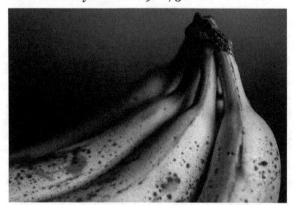

79. Coconut And Blueberries Ice Cream

Preparation time: 5 mins

Cooking time: 0 mins

Servings: 4

Ingredients

1/4 Cup Coconut Cream

1 Tbsp. Maple Syrup

¼ Cup Coconut Flour

1 Cup Blueberries

¼ Cup Blueberries For Topping

Directions

Put ingredients into food processor and mix well on high speed.

Pour mixture in silicon molds and freeze in freezer for about 2-4 hours.

Once balls are set remove from freezer.

Top with berries.

Serve cold and enjoy!

Nutrition: Protein: 3% 4 kcal Fat: 40% 60 kcal Carbohydrates: 57% 86 kcal

80. Peach Crockpot Pudding

Preparation time: 15 mins

Cooking time: 4 hours

Servings: 6

Ingredients

2 Cups Sliced Peaches

1/4 Cup Maple Syrup

/2 Tsp. Cinnamon Powder

2 Cups Coconut Milk

For Serving

½ Cup Coconut Cream

1 Oz. Coconut Flakes

Directions

Lightly grease the crockpot and place peaches in the bottom.

Add maple syrup, cinnamon powder and milk.

Cover and cook on high for 4 hours.

Once cooked remove from crockpot.

For serving pour coconut cream.

Top with coconut flakes.

Serve and enjoy!

Nutrition: Protein: 3% 11 kcal Fat: 61% 230 kcal Carbohydrates: 36% 133 kcal

81.Raspberries & Cream Ice Cream

Preparation time: 5 mins

Cooking time: 0 mins

Servings: 4

Ingredients

2 Cups Raspberries

8 Oz. Coconut Cream

2 Tbsps. Coconut Flour

1 Tsp Maple Syrup

4-8 Raspberries For Filling

Directions

Mix all ingredients in food processor and blend until well combined.

Spoon mixture into silicone mold and with raspberries and freeze for about 4 hours.

Remove balls from freezer and pop them out of the molds.

Serve immediately and enjoy!

Nutrition: Protein: 5% 12 kcal Fat: 69% 170 kcal Carbohydrates: 26% 63 kcal

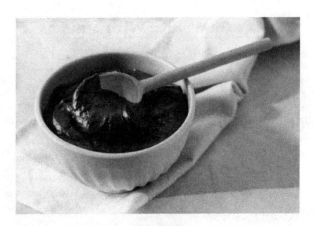

82. Healthy Chocolate Mousse

Preparation time: 5 mins

Cooking time: 0 mins

Servings: 2

Ingredients

1/2 Cup Coconut Milk

1 Tsp. Maple Syrup

1-3 Tbsps. Cocoa Powder

Pinch Instant Coffee

2 Tbsps. Coconut Cream

Blackberries For Topping

Directions

Heat up coconut milk and maple syrup until it just begins to simmer.

Add cocoa and coffee in milk mixture.

Add cream to same mixture and whip until relatively stiff peaks form.

Transfer to a serving glass.

Chill the mousse in freezer for 2-3 hours.

Top with some berries and spoon of coconut cream.

Enjoy!

Nutrition: Protein: 3% 7 kcal Fat: 83% 163 kcal Carbohydrates: 13% 26 kcal

83.   Coconut Rice With Mangos

Preparation time: 15 mins

Cooking time: 40 mins

Servings: 6

Ingredients

2 Cups Coconut Milk

1-1/2 Cups Coconut Flakes

1/4 Cup Maple Syrup

1 Mango Sliced

Directions

Heat saucepan over high heat.

Add coconut milk and bring it to boil.

Stir in coconut flakes and maple syrup.

Cover and cook on low heat for about 15 minutes or until liquid is completely dried.

Pour coconut rice in plate.

Serve with mango slice and enjoy.

Nutrition: Protein: 3% 8 kcal Fat: 69% 185 kcal Carbohydrates: 28% 75 kcal

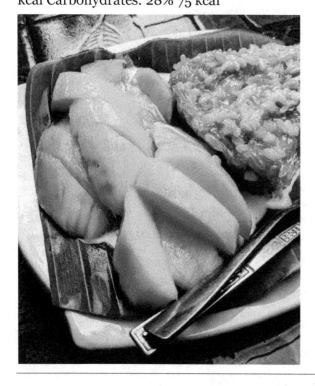

84.   Nori Snack Rolls

Preparation Time: 5 minutes

Cooking time: 10 minutes

Servings: 4 rolls

Ingredients

2 tablespoons almond, cashew, peanut, or others nut butter

2 tablespoons tamari, or soy sauce

4 standard nori sheets

1 mushroom, sliced

1 tablespoon pickled ginger

½ cup grated carrots

Directions

Preparing the Ingredients.

Preheat the oven to 350°F.

Mix together the nut butter and tamari until smooth and very thick. Lay out a nori sheet, rough side up, the long way.

Spread a thin line of the tamari mixture on the far end of the nori sheet, from side to side. Lay the mushroom slices, ginger, and carrots in a line at the other end (the end closest to you).

Fold the vegetables inside the nori, rolling toward the tahini mixture, which will seal the roll. Repeat to make 4 rolls.

Put on a baking sheet and bake for 8 to 10 minutes, or until the rolls are slightly browned and crispy at the ends. Let the rolls cool for a few minutes, then slice each roll into 3 smaller pieces.

Nutrition: Calories: 79; Total fat: 5g; Carbs: 6g; Fiber: 2g; Protein: 4g

85. Risotto Bites

Preparation Time: 15 minutes

Cooking time: 20 minutes

Servings: 12 bites

Ingredients

½ cup panko bread crumbs

1 teaspoon paprika

1 teaspoon chipotle powder or ground cayenne pepper

1½ cups cold Green Pea Risotto

Nonstick cooking spray

Directions

Preparing the Ingredients.

Preheat the oven to 425°F.

Line a baking sheet with parchment paper.

On a large plate, combine the panko, paprika, and chipotle powder. Set aside.

Roll 2 tablespoons of the risotto into a ball.

Gently roll in the bread crumbs, and place on the prepared baking sheet. Repeat to make a total of 12 balls.

Spritz the tops of the risotto bites with nonstick cooking spray and bake for 15 to 20 minutes, until they begin to brown. Cool completely before storing in a large airtight container in a single layer (add a piece of parchment paper for a second layer) or in a plastic freezer bag.

Nutrition: Calories: 100; Fat: 2g; Protein: 6g; Carbohydrates: 17g; Fiber: 5g; Sugar: 2g; Sodium: 165 mg

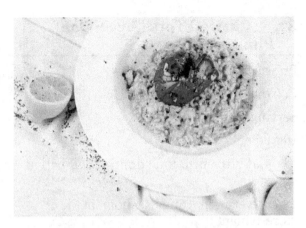

86. Jicama and Guacamole

Preparation Time: 15 minutes

Cooking time: 0 minutes

Servings: 4

Ingredients

juice of 1 lime, or 1 tablespoon prepared lime juice

2 hass avocados, peeled, pits removed, and cut into cubes

½ teaspoon sea salt

½ red onion, minced

1 garlic clove, minced

¼ cup chopped cilantro (optional)

1 jicama bulb, peeled and cut into matchsticks

Directions

Preparing the Ingredients.

In a medium bowl, squeeze the lime juice over the top of the avocado and sprinkle with salt.

Lightly mash the avocado with a fork. Stir in the onion, garlic, and cilantro, if using.

Serve with slices of jicama to dip in guacamole.

To store, place plastic wrap over the bowl of guacamole and refrigerate. The guacamole will keep for about 2 days.

87. Curried Tofu "Egg Salad" Pitas

Preparation Time: 15 minutes

Cooking time: 0 minutes

Servings: 4 sandwiches

Ingredients

1 pound extra-firm tofu, drained and patted dry

1/2 cup vegan mayonnaise, homemade or store-bought

1/4 cup chopped mango chutney, homemade or store-bought

2 teaspoons Dijon mustard

1 tablespoon hot or mild curry powder

1 teaspoon salt

1/8 teaspoon ground cayenne

3/4 cup shredded carrots

2 celery ribs, minced

1/4 cup minced red onion

8 small Boston or other soft lettuce leaves

4 (7-inch) whole wheat pita breads, halved

Directions

Crumble the tofu and place it in a large bowl. Add the mayonnaise, chutney, mustard, curry powder, salt, and cayenne, and stir well until thoroughly mixed.

Add the carrots, celery, and onion and stir to combine. Refrigerate for 30 minutes to allow the flavors to blend.

Tuck a lettuce leaf inside each pita pocket, spoon some tofu mixture on top of the lettuce, and serve.

88. Garden Salad Wraps

Preparation Time: 15 minutes

Cooking time: 10 minutes

Servings: 4 wraps

Ingredients

6 tablespoons olive oil

1 pound extra-firm tofu, drained, patted dry, and cut into 1/2-inch strips

1 tablespoon soy sauce

1/4 cup apple cider vinegar

1 teaspoon yellow or spicy brown mustard

1/2 teaspoon salt

1/4 teaspoon freshly ground black pepper

3 cups shredded romaine lettuce

3 ripe Roma tomatoes, finely chopped

1 large carrot, shredded

1 medium English cucumber, peeled and chopped

1/3 cup minced red onion

1/4 cup sliced pitted green olives

4 (10-inch) whole-grain flour tortillas or lavash flatbread

Directions

In a large skillet, heat 2 tablespoons of the oil over medium heat. Add the tofu and cook until golden brown, about 10 minutes. Sprinkle with soy sauce and set aside to cool.

In a small bowl, combine the vinegar, mustard, salt, and pepper with the remaining 4 tablespoons oil, stirring to blend well. Set aside.

In a large bowl, combine the lettuce, tomatoes, carrot, cucumber, onion, and olives. Pour on the dressing and toss to coat.

To assemble wraps, place 1 tortilla on a work surface and spread with about one-quarter of the salad. Place a few strips of tofu on the tortilla and roll up tightly. Slice in half 76.

89. Tamari Toasted Almonds

Preparation Time: 2 minutes

Cooking time: 8 minutes

Servings: ½ cup

Ingredients

½ cup raw almonds, or sunflower seeds

2 tablespoons tamari, or soy sauce

1 teaspoon toasted sesame oil

Directions

Preparing the Ingredients.

Heat a dry skillet to medium-high heat, then add the almonds, stirring very frequently to keep them from burning. Once the almonds are toasted, 7 to 8 minutes for almonds, or 3 to 4 minutes for sunflower seeds, pour the tamari and sesame oil into the hot skillet and stir to coat.

You can turn off the heat, and as the almonds cool the tamari mixture will stick to and dry on the nuts.

Per Serving (1 tablespoon) Calories: 89; Total fat: 8g; Carbs: 3g; Fiber: 2g; Protein: 4g

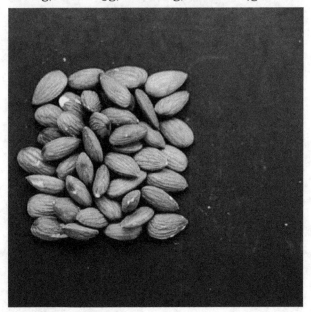

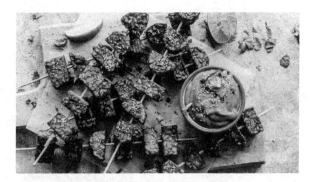

90. Avocado And Tempeh Bacon Wraps

Preparation Time: 10 minutes

Cooking time: 8 minutes

Servings: 4 wraps

Ingredients

2 tablespoons olive oil

8 ounces tempeh bacon, homemade or store-bought

4 (10-inch) soft flour tortillas or lavash flatbread

¼ cup vegan mayonnaise, homemade or store-bought

4 large lettuce leaves

2 ripe Hass avocados, pitted, peeled, and cut into ¼-inch slices

1 large ripe tomato, cut into ¼-inch slices

Directions

In a large skillet, heat the oil over medium heat. Add the tempeh bacon and cook until browned on both sides, about 8 minutes. Remove from the heat and set aside.

Place 1 tortilla on a work surface. Spread with some of the mayonnaise and one-fourth of the lettuce and tomatoes.

Pit, peel, and thinly slice the avocado and place the slices on top of the tomato. Add the reserved tempeh bacon and roll up tightly. Repeat with remaining Ingredients and serve.

91. Kale Chips

Preparation Time: 5 minutes

Cooking time: 25 minutes

Servings: 2

Ingredients

1 large bunch kale

1 tablespoon extra-virgin olive oil

½ teaspoon chipotle powder

½ teaspoon smoked paprika

¼ teaspoon salt

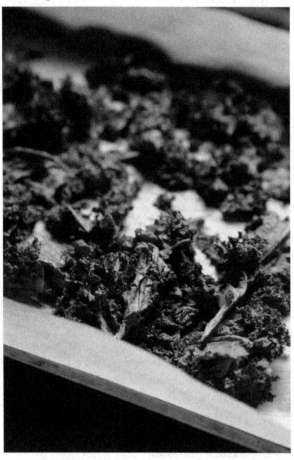

Directions

Preparing the Ingredients.

Preheat the oven to 275°F.

Line a large baking sheet with parchment paper. In a large bowl, stem the kale and tear it into bite-size pieces. Add the olive oil, chipotle powder, smoked paprika, and salt.

Toss the kale with tongs or your hands, coating each piece well.

Spread the kale over the parchment paper in a single layer.

Bake for 25 minutes, turning halfway through, until crisp.

Cool for 10 to 15 minutes before dividing and storing in 2 airtight containers.

Nutrition: Calories: 144; Fat: 7g; Protein: 5g; Carbohydrates: 18g; Fiber: 3g; Sugar: 0g; Sodium: 363mg

21-Day Meal Plan

Day	Breakfast	Entrées	Soup , Salad, & Sides	Smoothie
1	Tasty Oatmeal Muffins	Black Bean Dip	Spinach Soup with Dill and Basil	Fruity Smoothie
2	Omelet with Chickpea Flour	Cannellini Bean Cashew Dip	Coconut Watercress Soup	Energizing Ginger Detox Tonic
3	White Sandwich Bread	Cauliflower Popcorn	Coconut Watercress Soup	Warm Spiced Lemon Drink
4	A Toast to Remember	Cinnamon Apple Chips with Dip	Coconut Watercress Soup	Soothing Ginger Tea Drink
5	Tasty Panini	Crunchy Asparagus Spears	Cauliflower Spinach Soup	Nice Spiced Cherry Cider
6	Tasty Oatmeal and Carrot Cake	Cucumber Bites with Chive and Sunflower Seeds	Avocado Mint Soup	Fragrant Spiced Coffee
7	Onion & Mushroom Tart with a Nice Brown Rice Crust	Garlicky Kale Chips	Creamy Squash Soup	Tangy Spiced Cranberry Drink
8	Perfect Breakfast Shake	Hummus-stuffed Baby Potatoes	Cucumber Edamame Salad	Warm Pomegranate Punch
9	Beet Gazpacho	Homemade Trail Mix	Best Broccoli Salad	Rich Truffle Hot Chocolate
10	Vegetable Rice	Nut Butter Maple Dip	Rainbow Orzo Salad	Ultimate Mulled Wine
11	Courgette Risotto	Oven Baked Sesame Fries	Broccoli Pasta Salad	Pleasant Lemonade
12	Country Breakfast Cereal	Pumpkin Orange Spice Hummus	Eggplant & Roasted Tomato Farro Salad	Pineapple, Banana & Spinach Smoothie
13	Oatmeal Fruit Shake	Quick English Muffin Mexican Pizzas	Garden Patch Sandwiches on Multigrain Bread	Kale & Avocado Smoothie
14	Amaranth Banana Breakfast Porridge	Quinoa Trail Mix Cups	Garden Salad Wraps	Coconut & Strawberry Smoothie

15	Green Ginger Smoothie	Black Bean Dip	Marinated Mushroom Wraps	Pumpkin Chia Smoothie
16	Orange Dream Creamsicle	Cannellini Bean Cashew Dip	Tamari Toasted Almonds	Cantaloupe Smoothie Bowl
17	Strawberry Limeade	Cauliflower Popcorn	Nourishing Whole-Grain Porridge	Berry & Cauliflower Smoothie
18	Peanut Butter and Jelly Smoothie	Cinnamon Apple Chips with Dip	Pungent Mushroom Barley Risotto	Green Mango Smoothie
19	Banana Almond Granola	Crunchy Asparagus Spears	Spinach Soup with Dill and Basil	Chia Seed Smoothie
20	Tasty Oatmeal Muffins	Cucumber Bites with Chive and Sunflower Seeds	Coconut Watercress Soup	Mango Smoothie
21	Omelet with Chickpea Flour	Garlicky Kale Chips	Coconut Watercress Soup	Fruity Smoothie

Conclusions

I want to thank you once again for choosing this book. I hope it proved to be an informative read.

A plant-based diet primarily involves consuming foods that are entirely derived from plants. The primary idea of this diet is to increase your consumption of healthy and wholesome foods while eliminating processed foods. By now, you have realized the various benefits this diet offers. By increasing your consumption of the different plant-based foods mentioned in this book, you can attain your weight-loss objectives, improve your overall health, and reduce your risk of developing several serious illnesses.

Now, you just need to stock up your pantry with the required ingredients mentioned in the food list in this book. By concentrating on certain anti-inflammatory foods, you can tackle inflammation effectively. All the recipes given in this book are easy to prepare, tasty and healthy. Use the various plant-based alternatives to the regular foods you consume, and you won't feel like you're missing out on anything.

If you're excited to get started with a plant-based diet, use the 21-day meal plan provided in this book to plan out all your meals. Cooking has never been this easy! You don't need to compromise your taste buds for the sake of your health. By following a plant-based diet, you can effectively eat your way to better health.

So, what are you waiting for? Let's get rustling in the kitchen.

Thank you, and all the best.